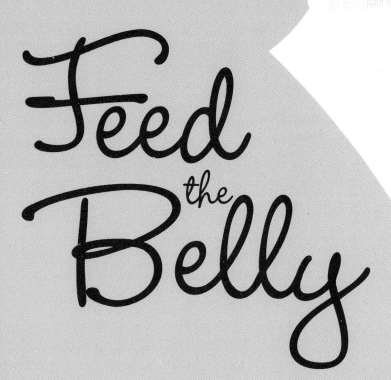

Feed the Belly

The Pregnant Mom's Healthy Eating Guide

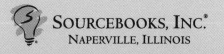

SOURCEBOOKS, INC.
NAPERVILLE, ILLINOIS

Frances Largeman-Roth, RD
Foreword by Robin Miller

Published by Sourcebooks, Inc.
P.O. Box 4410, Naperville, Illinois 60567-4410
(630) 961-3900
Fax: (630) 961-2168
www.sourcebooks.com

Library of Congress Cataloging-in-Publication Data

Largeman-Roth, Frances.
  Feed the belly : the pregnant mom's healthy eating guide / Frances Largeman-Roth.
      p. cm.
  1. Pregnancy—Nutritional aspects. I. Title.

RG559.L37 2009
618.2'42—dc22

2008038969

Printed and bound in the United States of America.

UGI 10 9 8 7 6 5 4 3 2

Praise for *Feed the Belly*

"*Feed the Belly* is overdue! If you are pregnant or living with someone who is, you will find this book to be invaluable to the pregnancy. It has knowledgeable information, great anecdotes, recipes and tips for navigating the challenges and surprises of pregnancy. *Feed the Belly* can help in creating a happier, healthier journey for the whole family."

—Cat Cora, the first female Iron Chef and author of
Cooking from the Hip

"Finally a comprehensive, fun-to-read, realistic guide to eating well when you are expecting. I wish this book were out when I was pregnant!"

—Ellie Krieger, MS, RD, author of *The Food You Crave* and host of
Food Network's *Healthy Appetite*

"*Feed the Belly* is a terrific one-stop shop for any mom-to-be who wants to eat well and feel well right up to the big event and even after. Frances Largeman-Roth gives you the keep-it-real version on how to eat and how to deal with pregnancy. This is a great read for any expectant mom—and even dads can learn something!"

—Keith-Thomas Ayoob, EdD, RD, associate pediatrics professor,
Albert Einstein College of Medicine

*For my mother. Thanks for eating your vegetables
and getting me to love them, too.
Your spirit and determination never cease
to inspire those around you.*

Contents

Foreword

When Frances Largeman-Roth asked me to write the foreword for this book, I was thrilled and honored. Frances and I have known each other and worked together for many years. When she mentioned she was writing a comprehensive yet easy-to-understand cookbook for moms-to-be, I was on board in two seconds. Let's face it: Pregnant women tackle the scary work of eating right every minute of every day they're sporting the bump!

I have two little ones myself, and during both pregnancies I spent countless hours at the bookstore searching through dozens of nutrition and cookbooks for just the *right* book. The sad truth—that time would have been better spent working on the baby's room, because I often left empty-handed. Why? Because most books contained more data than I learned when I was in graduate school, pursuing a master's degree in nutrition! I'm a nutrition professional, and if *I* can't find a good book on the subject, there's something wrong with this picture. Thankfully, Frances has put together all the necessary information for expectant mothers in one concise package.

Both of my pregnancies were pretty easy, but whether yours is trouble-free or challenging, Frances navigates you through the dizzying maze of nutrition advice we're bombarded with every day. Her guidance is current and sound, and she provides the science to back it up. Best of all, Frances holds your hand through the entire process—from the earliest weeks to the post-birth quest for fitting into your skinny jeans.

It's important to think about what you're eating when you can't stomach much, and that's why I love "Chapter 2: Baby Bonuses and Momma Must-Haves." The particulars Frances gives on important pregnancy-related vitamins and minerals are precise, clear, and loaded with great food examples that include portion sizes. Frances also tackles some current quandaries, such as the safety of plastic bottles and the use of essential oils during a tension-relieving massage.

If you're like most women, you're probably dealing with some pretty odd cravings. Frances does a great job of explaining the ins and outs of food cravings and aversions in "Chapter 3: She's Gotta Have It." With both pregnancies, I experienced the *exact same* cravings. Don't hate me, but they were pretty healthy. My number one "gotta-have-it" food was lentils—namely, Progresso Lentil Soup. I craved it with both boys for forty solid weeks each. Sometimes the desire was so strong that I'd eat the soup, straight from the can, in the car while still in the grocery store parking lot—thank goodness for those pop-top lids! As for aversions, I struggled with seafood. One of my favorite foods is shrimp, but while I was pregnant, just the thought of those cute little crustaceans made my stomach churn. Thankfully, the aversion disappeared once my boys were born.

Some well-intentioned pregnancy books recommend enough "must-have" foods to make your head spin. "Chapter 4: The Pregnancy Pantry" is comprehensive without being daunting, listing good-for-you, everyday items that are readily available. Frances highlights which foods you should choose, and *why* you should choose them. She also discusses various gadgets that make life easier in the kitchen by streamlining the cooking process. That's so important during pregnancy, because you're often too tired or too busy to "labor" over preparing a meal (pun intended!).

Even if you've never contemplated it before, pregnancy often ignites the pro/con debate over organic foods. In "Chapter 6: The Big O (Organic, That Is)," Frances stresses the importance of certain organic ingredients while illustrating which foods pack the biggest nutrient punch. She also lists some foods that may help prevent childhood asthma.

In "Chapter 7: Go Fish," you'll find excellent, current information about which fish should become pregnancy staples. Not a fish-eater? Or dealing with the same aversion I had? Frances provides ideas for foods that contain similar essential nutrients.

I was lucky…I didn't struggle with morning sickness (just a little queasy for the first twelve weeks). For those of you who are suffering through it, check out Frances's tips in "Chapter 9: Belly Blues—Morning Sickness Survival Guide."

If you stick to a meat-, dairy-, or even wheat-free diet, Frances provides fabulous information on choosing the foods that'll ensure you and your baby get the nutrients you need.

And then there's the weight gain/weight loss issue. I gained more than 40 pounds with each boy and I didn't fret one bit. I knew I would get back to my fighting weight by establishing a healthy eating and exercise routine (in between changing diapers and breast-feeding, of course). Frances gives easy-to-follow guidelines for weight gain and then follows it up with a chapter on prenatal exercise. She even includes great advice on where to find comfortable and cute maternity fitness clothes!

If all this useful information isn't enough, just wait until you try the recipes! There are more than sixty-five recipes in this book. You can select a meal based on your cravings (sweet, meaty, salty/savory, spicy, or thirst-quenching). The way things are cross-referenced, you can also look up a recipe based on major nutrients, ideal for those days when you're trying to pack in more iron and want to dodge that burger. The nutritional analysis that goes with each recipe is incredibly useful, and I especially like the **Baby Bonuses**, tips about particular nutrients in the dishes that are necessary for your baby's growth.

The bottom line? Frances has tons of experience writing for women, so she speaks in a language we can all understand. Shop no further! You've found the one book you need to get you through this pregnancy—and beyond. Now you'll have plenty of time for that baby room.

—**Robin Miller**, cookbook author, nutritionist, and host of Food Network's *Quick Fix Meals with Robin Miller*

Acknowledgments

A huge thanks to my agents, Adina Kahn and Jane Dystel of Dystel and Goderich, for their never-ending enthusiasm for this project. And a second big thanks to my incredible editor at Sourcebooks, Inc., Shana Drehs. You believed in *Feed the Belly* from the start and helped me mold and shape it until it was just right. Thanks to the rest of the creative crew at Sourcebooks, too. And to Robin Miller, a huge thanks for your enthusiasm, support, and mom-insight.

I'm also immensely grateful to all the experts who shared their time and insights with me: Dr. Mark Messina; Dr. Emily Oken; Dr. Margaret Someral; Steve Otwell, PhD; Dr. Marlene Reid; Shelley Feist; Miriam Erick, MS, RD, CDE; and Sara Ivanhoe. And to all of my chef and cookbook author friends who contributed recipes—your good taste is greatly appreciated: Mark Bittman, Cat Cora, Gale Gand, David Guas, Peggy Knickerbocker, Emily Luchetti, Steven Raichlen, Joanne Weir, and Grace Young.

I'd be remiss if I didn't thank all the ladies who shared their stories of crazy cravings and morning-sickness misery with me. You know who you are. And I never would have gotten this off the ground without the stories and support of my two favorite women, my mom and my sister Elizabeth.

Extra-special thanks to my amazingly understanding and patient husband Jon, who never complained that the book took up my weekends, nights, and vacations. I couldn't have done it without you, Sweetie.

Introduction

Chances are, if you're reading this book, you've recently received some seriously exciting news. Congratulations! Or maybe you've just gotten started on a journey to prepare your body for pregnancy.

It's a fabulous time to have a bun in the oven. Being a mom-to-be is no longer something to hide. It's a state to celebrate, a time to embrace the changes going on in your body. In fact, our entire society seems to be baby-crazed, with the dietary lapses and stiletto-wearing habits of celebrity moms-to-be being closely watched. But you don't need to follow the bump watches in the pages of *Us Weekly*—you've got your own bump to consider. The next nine months are going to be a wild ride, including hunger pangs mixed with indigestion and moments of utter bliss tossed together with extreme fatigue and nausea. Through it all, the most important things on your mind will be your baby's health.

Like most expectant moms, you probably have a lot of questions about how to ensure the best health possible for your baby. Science in general and prenatal medicine specifically are changing constantly, and the advice your mom got about what to eat and how to exercise when pregnant is much different from what you'll get from your doctor today. *Feed the Belly* gives you the latest information on everything relating to food, nutrition, and living a healthy lifestyle during your entire pregnancy. You'll find an eating guide for those nine months that helps you navigate through morning sickness, crazy cravings, and endless quandaries over what's safe to put in your mouth. You'll also find more than sixty-five recipes, because aside from hiring your own personal chef—a girl can dream, right?—the best way for you to make sure you're getting what you need is to prepare most of your own meals and snacks (and get your hubby to pitch in, too).

Life doesn't necessarily slow down just because you're expecting, and that's where I come in. As a registered dietitian with a decade of experience creating nutrition information and developing recipes specifically targeted to women, I know what it takes to create a dish that's healthy, delicious, and really hits the spot. As *Health* magazine's senior food and nutrition editor since 2004, it's been my task to come up with mouthwatering dishes that keep busy women satisfied *and* able to fit into little black dresses.

Plus, I'm picky as all get out, and when I started on my own quest to become a mom, I quickly found there wasn't anything on the shelves that really spoke to me. All of the so-called pregnancy cookbooks and nutrition manuals contained recipes that were about as exciting as the early-bird special at Sizzler. Come on, people! Pregnant women still have taste buds. The recipes I created for the book had to meet my high standards for taste and crave-worthiness, and since I was pregnant while I was working on them, I was the *perfect* guinea pig.

Going through my first pregnancy while writing this book gave me a front-line view of what advice is realistic, and what is a lot of well-meaning hooey. Normally, I'm a fruit, yogurt, and whole-grain kind of girl in the morning, but during my first trimester, I was all about egg-and-cheese break-fast sandwiches with ketchup, bags of salty pretzels, and jugs of Orangina. (I discovered that when you're pregnant and trying to get through the work-day, a settled stomach often outweighs a perfectly balanced meal.) But I also found ways to get around my lust for salty carbs and sneak in some fruit and veggies when I was feeling more steady. Little swaps—like an organic cheese stick instead of my usual yogurt—helped me fit in calcium and protein while satisfying my salty cravings.

The *Feed the Belly* recipes I've created (starting on page 150) range from easy, cooling smoothies to healthier versions of comfort foods like chicken pot pie and burgers. All are easy to make, and I've included tips for even easier and faster variations. Every recipe has a complete nutritional analysis, and I've made note of particularly important nutrients for your baby's growth as **Baby Bonuses**. Goodies for you are designated with a **Momma Must-Have** note.

If you're on the road to getting pregnant, turn to "Chapter 1: Trying for a Bump." You'll find lots of tips for foods and vitamins to add to your diet (and those to avoid) in order to make your body a welcome home for a little one. If you're already pregnant, you can dive right into "Chapter 2: Baby Bonuses and Momma Must-Haves."

What's more, *Feed the Belly* is the first book to organize recipes by the strongest pregnancy cravings. Even if you had willpower of steel before you became pregnant, once you're expecting you might find yourself pulled by an inner magnet to fast-food restaurants, bakeries, ice-cream parlors, and steakhouses. Science is still fuzzy on whether food cravings during pregnancy indicate nutrient needs or deficiencies, but one thing's for sure—when a craving strikes, there's almost nothing you can do but give in to it. For some women, it's a greasy cheeseburger at 8 a.m., while others hanker for healthier fare, like kiwi or celery.

The good news: It's fine to succumb to those nacho and ice-cream cone desires once in a while, but you also want to make sure your baby is getting the nutrients she needs to develop, and you're getting the energy *you* need to feel your best. I designed the recipes in this book around crave-worthy foods, such as mac 'n' cheese, and then added a few secret ingredients to boost the good-for-you profile and help you cover the bases on important nutrients like folic acid, calcium, and iron. At the end of the day, all the recipes had to pass the all-important taste test. If food doesn't bring you enjoyment, what's the point?

Want something sweet? Turn to page 157 for a dozen mouthwatering choices (like Peach and Blackberry Crumble, for example) that tap into the most common pregnancy cravings for sweets: chocolatey, citrusy, creamy, fruity, and salty/sweet. Dying for something salty and savory? How about Mediterranean Barley Salad or Miso Pretty Soup?

Not craving anything in particular…or maybe your doctor told you to get more iron? You can also look up recipes by major nutrient, such as protein, omega-3 fatty acids, or calcium.

You'll also see **Belly Tips** sprinkled throughout the book. These are extra-important notes on how to boost your nutrition—little nuggets of information that you usually only get from your best girlfriends, like how to trick yourself into drinking more water or the best time of day to take your prenatal vitamin.

To keep you on track from morning till night, I've designed a seven-day eating plan that you can tear out and take with you for guidance on-the-go. Just turn to the back of the book and rip it out. How cool is that?

A girl has to lean on her friends for a little help once in a while, so I decided to reach out and ask a few chef and cookbook author pals to pitch in a favorite recipe. You'll find out what celeb pastry chef Gale Gand craved during her pregnancy with twins, as well as Food Network Iron Chef Cat Cora's sure cure for meaty cravings. Bestselling cookbook author Mark Bittman shares a belly-friendly recipe that perfectly illustrates his minimalist style of cooking.

Hectic schedules mean that most of us are dining out often—as much as three times a week—so I'll also give you the skinny on how to make smart choices at restaurants and even fast-food places (yep, there *are* some good picks out there). Plus, regular snacking will become your friend, so check out my list of go-to **Momma Munchies** on page 140.

Beyond just what to eat, other pregnancy worries might start creeping up on you. Anxiety over *E. coli*-tainted sprouts and listeriosis in deli meat may be on your mind, but they needn't keep you up at night. On page xxi, you'll find a cheat sheet of the top ten foods to avoid and the top ten foods to embrace. I know that doing what's best without going overboard can seem daunting, so look to "Chapter 14: Germ Patrol" to learn everything you need to know to stay germ-free without living in a bubble.

You'll be happy to know that you can still sweat it out on the treadmill and keep up with your Pilates classes. You just need to learn how to do it with a baby on board, and there are plenty of tips on doing just that in "Chapter 12: Sweating for Two." Plus, there's a bonus series of yoga poses from yoga master Sara Ivanhoe that will help you restore your energy when you're feeling less than perky.

There's a lot to think about during these next nine months. Some of it is daunting (blood tests) and some of it is absolutely thrilling (hearing your baby's heartbeat for the first time). You've probably already discovered that once the word is out about your upcoming bundle of joy, you're inundated with advice from everyone from well-meaning grannies to bossy sales girls. They'll fill your mind so full of conflicting information on what you can and can't eat that you'll be ready to forfeit your whisk and cutting board forever. The reality is that eating for pregnancy is pretty much like regular healthy eating, with a few caveats for making what goes in your body as safe as possible.

Let's face it: You're not going to do everything right 100 percent of the time. I'm a perfectionist, so it was hard for me to wrap my brain around that idea at first. Look at it this way—if you eat right 90 percent of the time, you're doing a pretty fantastic job. It's good practice for motherhood, when you're striving to do everything right but often end up feeling inadequate. Do the best you can, and don't let anyone make you feel bad if you're not baking your own flax-spelt-quinoa bread or making your own sheep's-milk yogurt.

After all, any healthy choices you make will be beneficial, and not only for your baby! As an added bonus, getting savvy about healthy eating now means it'll be easier to get active, lose the baby weight, and fit into your skinny jeans post-pregnancy. (Boy, wouldn't that be nice?) Plus, studies show that kids tend to develop a taste for the foods their moms eat during pregnancy and breast-feeding.[1] Wouldn't you love it if your child ended up preferring peaches and peas to pound cake?

Here's another reason to load up on the healthy stuff. A diet in the Mediterranean style—low in animal protein and saturated fats and rich in fruits, vegetables, monounsaturated fats, legumes, seafood, and whole grains—helps lower your kid's risk of asthma. One study that examined the elementary school–aged children of Spanish moms who had eaten a Mediterranean diet while they were pregnant found that the kids were less likely to develop asthma or allergies. The researchers think that seafood and vegetables played the biggest roles in protecting these kids.[2] (You, too, can go Med with my Mediterranean Barley Salad, on page 213.)

Even though many of your pregnancy experiences will be beyond your control (hello, hemorrhoids and acne) and will cause you lots of added anxiety, what you choose to feed your body with is (thankfully) completely in your hands. With a little planning, it's really quite easy to do, too. This book will help you feed your cravings *and* get your baby the nutrients she needs. I also make a solemn promise that you won't find any recipes for fruit-juice sweetened cookies…just good, old-fashioned recipes and wholesome ingredients that taste really freaking good. (Pssst…you *can* eat cookies for breakfast once in a while, but only if they're my Oh, Baby! Breakfast Cookies, on page 183.)

So take a deep breath, bring your appetite, and take care of that growing belly.

Feed the Belly's Top 10 Things to Avoid and Top 10 Things to Enjoy

What to Avoid

1. **Alcohol**.

2. **Tobacco** (weed, too!).

3. **Caffeine**; limit it as much as possible. That includes energy drinks that contain natural forms of caffeine, like guarana, yerba mate, or ginseng.

4. **Unpasteurized (raw) milk, juice, and other beverages.**

5. **Unpasteurized soft cheeses**, such as Brie, Camembert, blue cheese, feta, and queso fresco.

6. **Processed meats**, such as lunch meat, hot dogs (unless they're steaming hot), lox, meat spreads, and pâté.

7. **Raw foods, including meat, fish** (sushi), **shellfish, eggs** (sorry, honey, that includes raw cookie dough), and **sprouts** (including alfalfa, mung, clover, and radish).

8. **Fish that are high in mercury** (cooked or uncooked), such as swordfish, tilefish, king mackerel, and shark.

9. **Herbal supplements**.

10. **Artificial sweeteners** (unless you're diabetic).

What to Enjoy

1. **Folic acid-rich foods**, such as fortified cereal, lentils, edamame, spinach, asparagus, and citrus fruits.

2. **Iron-packed foods**, such as beef, bison, chicken, eggs, salmon, Swiss chard, dried apricots, and tofu.

3. **Protein**, which can be found in lean meat, poultry, seafood, soy-based foods, nuts, low-fat dairy products, and quinoa.

4. **Omega-3 fatty acids**, which are plentiful in salmon, tuna, enriched eggs, walnuts, and flax seeds.

5. **Choline**, a nutrient important for baby's brain health, which you'll get in eggs, soy-based foods, pork chops, and cauliflower.

6. **Calcium** to build strong bones and teeth, found in milk, yogurt, cheese, spinach, and broccoli.

7. **Vitamin B$_{12}$**, a vitamin found in cooked clams, beef liver, fortified cereal, trout, salmon, and beef.

8. **Vitamin D**, a critical vitamin that's abundant in eggs, salmon, sardines, fortified milk, and good old sunshine.

9. **Vitamin C**, which you'll get in strawberries, red bell peppers, and citrus fruits.

10. **Zinc**, a mineral that you can get in fortified cereal, beef, pork, chicken, yogurt, beans, and cashews.

Chapter One

Trying for a Bump

Note: If you've already got a growing belly, move on to
"Chapter 2: Baby Bonuses and Momma Must-Haves"!

Y ou've done the research. You know that after your twenty-seventh birthday, your chances of conceiving start to drop, and suddenly getting pregnant becomes like getting into an Ivy League school—you've got to be seriously on your game. Many of us (including me) are in this boat now, since one in five women today have their first child after the age of thirty-five.[1] If you've been working on having a baby for a while, you've probably been religiously charting your cycle, peeing on ovulation prediction sticks (oh…how romantic), and buying pregnancy tests in bulk. But you may not have thought all that much about what you're eating and drinking.

There are no magical fertility foods, but you can change your diet to improve your chances. Making some simple tweaks to your diet three months (or more) before trying to conceive is a smart idea. The main goal is to stay healthy, because a healthy body is a much more welcoming place for a hot date between egg and sperm.

Fertility Helpers

The number one change you'll want to make is to include more **folate-rich foods**. Eat more fortified cereals, asparagus, lentils, oranges, orange juice, and everyone's fave, chicken livers. Check the label on the multivitamin you currently take, as you may already be getting enough folic acid. It should have at least 400 micrograms (mcg) in it. If not, add a supplement with that amount of folic acid. (Folic acid is the same thing as folate, but the latter comes from food sources.)

Folic acid is crucial for the proper development of the baby's neural tube (it covers the spinal cord), which is formed during the first month of pregnancy. Getting enough folic acid *before* you're pregnant helps prevent serious birth defects, such as spina bifida. It's the one thing you should change about your diet when you first start trying, anywhere from three months to one year before you and your partner get serious about making a baby. You have to make sure you're fully stocked up on folic acid, because you never know which month is going to be *the* month. Once you know you're pregnant, you should increase your intake of folic acid to 600 to 800 mcg per day.

Beyond the fact that you're protecting a new little life inside you, folic acid also seems to boost your chances of getting pregnant in the first place. Studies have shown that taking a multivitamin with 800 mcg of the vitamin for at least twenty-eight days pre-conception and two months post-conception increased fertility.[2]

In fact, you may want to start popping that folic-acid pill even earlier than the suggested three months before trying to conceive. A recent observational analysis of National Institutes of Health (NIH) folic acid supplementation reports found that women who began taking a supplement a full year before conception experienced 70 percent lower rates of *super*-early preterm delivery (twenty to twenty-eight weeks) and a 50 percent reduction in early preterm delivery (twenty-eight to thirty-two weeks).[3] The study examined only women who took supplements and did not consider dietary folate—but we know that doesn't hurt either. Even if it takes you awhile to get pregnant, don't worry about getting that extra 400 to 800 mcg of folic acid in the meantime—it'll help keep your heart healthy, too.

Iron-packed foods are also essential because once you're pregnant, Junior starts robbing you of your iron reserves. In addition, a 2006 study showed that women who took iron supplements had a lower risk of ovulatory infertility than women who didn't take supplements.[4] Consider taking an iron supplement or a multivitamin that contains the recommended daily allowance (RDA) of iron for women: 18 mg. You certainly don't need to eat meat at every meal, but try to get a few servings a week of lean beef, chicken, fish, and pork (each will have about 2 to 3 mg of iron). Raisins, spinach, kale, Swiss chard, fortified cereals, tofu, beans, and dried apricots are great vegetarian sources of iron. Just remember that the vegetarian form—which is also called non-heme iron—is not as easily absorbed by your body as iron that comes from animal sources. That's easy to fix: Just make sure you eat a vitamin C-rich food at the same time as an iron-rich one, as vitamin C helps your body absorb iron. Some easy combos: Mix some salsa with your black beans, have a glass of O.J. with your fortified cereal, or throw some strawberries into a spinach salad. But watch out for your beloved Starbucks—it interferes with your iron absorption. Both coffee and tea will reduce the amount of iron you absorb, so take that latte break (see below for how much coffee is too much) between your meals.

Get **good fats**, such as omega-3s, from salmon, flax seeds, walnuts, and enhanced foods. Numerous studies have shown that getting enough docosahexanoic acid, or DHA, which is a form of omega-3, is essential for the development of a baby's brain and nervous system. The Food and Drug Administration hasn't set a recommended daily value yet for omega-3 (it's currently reviewing the issue), but try to fit in a few servings a day. That's so much easier today, considering the wide variety of omega-3 fortified products—juice, milk, soy milk, and enhanced eggs—that are available. Monounsaturated fats from nuts, seeds, olive oil, olives, and avocados are easy additions to your diet, too. They help keep your heart healthy and increase absorption of the fat-soluble vitamins A, D, E, and K. Plus, fat is essential for the production of hormones, and *Lord knows* you need to be making plenty of those to get preggers.

Now's the time to load up on **antioxidant-rich fruits and veggies** like blueberries (and other berries), artichokes, pomegranates, apples, beans, and dried plums (aka prunes). Antioxidants scavenge free radicals in the body and prevent cell damage (think of free radicals as a twenty-two-year-old at the office jockeying to steal your job someday). Getting enough antioxidants will help fight wear and tear on all of your cells, including your fragile eggs. How do you know you're getting enough? If you eat a beige diet, you're most likely not getting your antioxidant fix. Basically, the brighter and deeper the color of your food, the better it is for you. So make like Betsey Johnson and go crazy with color at each meal. Even in the winter, when there's not a ton of good-looking fresh produce available, you can still get your antioxidant fix from frozen fruits and veggies (see page 42 in the pantry section for more about why frozen fruits and veggies are your friend). Juices are a great way to get antioxidants, too—just stick to a small 6-ounce glass, or else you might rack up some serious calories. Studies show that the top antioxidant juices are (in order): pomegranate, Concord grape, blueberry, black cherry, açai, cranberry, and orange.[5]

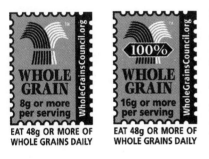

Be sure you switch out that flimsy white bread or wheat-colored bread for true whole-grain bread. Same goes for cereal and other grain products. **Whole grains** are not only a good source of fiber and minerals—they're also rich in antioxidants. Look for the words "whole wheat," "whole oats," or "whole barley" as the first ingredient on the ingredient list. Products that bear the Whole Grains Council's Whole Grain Stamp on the label have the good stuff. And these days, there are more whole-grain products than ever.

And get this—that ice-cream cone you're devouring on the sly may actually increase your chances of getting preggers! A Harvard study found that women who ate two or more servings of low-fat **dairy products** per week had a higher risk of ovulatory infertility, while women who consumed *full-fat* dairy (like ice cream and whole milk) with the same frequency had a lower incidence.[6] I'm not saying you should go to bed with an entire pint of cookies 'n' cream, but try to mix some of the regular stuff in with your low- and non-fat items. And it's healthier to go with low-fat (1%) than fat-free, because you need a certain amount of fat to absorb vitamins A and D, the fat-soluble vitamins found in fortified dairy products.

Other Goodies to Include When You're Trying

- **Eat Beta carotene-rich foods** like pumpkin, squash, sweet potatoes, and mango.

- Also enjoy vitamin-and-mineral-rich **whole grains** (oatmeal, brown rice, popcorn, and barley).

- Indulge in **enriched wheat products** like breakfast cereal and sandwich bread. Didn't I just tell you to choose whole grains a minute ago? Yes, but those great, grainy artisanal breads aren't enriched with folic acid, so eat a balance of both.

Belly Tip

Want a boy? Eat your Wheaties and throw some bananas on top. A study done by Britain's Oxford and Exeter Universities showed that women who had a high potassium intake and a higher calorie intake had more boys than women with reduced calorie diets and lower potassium intakes. There seemed to be a cereal link, too—59 percent of women who ate cereal each day had boys, compared to only 43 percent of women who ate less than a bowlful per week. But don't start digging into that stack of banana pancakes just yet—your chance of having a boy only increases by 5 percent.[7]

Fertility Foilers

A recent study showed that getting only 2 percent of your calories (a measly 40 calories, if you're eating about 2,000 per day) from **trans fat** (instead of healthier fats) can increase your risk of ovulatory infertility by up to 95 percent.[8] These days, it's easy to avoid trans fats for the most part. All labeled foods must list the amount of trans fat they contain. The tricky part is that, legally, products that have up to 0.5 gram per serving can list a trans fat content of zero. So, if you have four of those "trans fat-free" cookies instead of two, you could end up with an additional gram of trans fat—and since each gram of fat contains nine calories, you can see how the calories add up pretty fast. You can avoid trans fats completely by skipping products made with partially hydrogenated oils. Also, most fried food in restaurants is still cooked in partially hydrogenated oils, so lay off the French fries.

Keep happy hour to a minimum. There's nothing wrong with the occasional glass of wine, but **heavy drinking** (more than three drinks at a time) can mess up your menstrual cycle—ergo, your fertility.[9] Plus, it's well documented that alcohol causes various problems for a growing fetus, so if you're trying to get pregnant, minimize your alcohol consumption as much as possible, and once you get that positive test, nix the bar completely. To learn more about alcohol and pregnancy, turn to page 47.

Some researchers in the field of reproductive endocrinology believe that high insulin levels can interfere with normal ovulation. While the medical community hasn't fully established this, it makes sense that you'd want to avoid **erratic blood sugar levels**. Don't worry. This is actually pretty easy to do, and is smart anytime—not just when you want a baby. Just try to eat a balance of carbohydrates, protein, fiber, and fat at each meal…and no more skipping breakfast, ladies! Eat every four hours or so to keep your blood sugar level steady. When you go without eating for too long and become ravenous, it's nearly impossible to make good food choices (which is why you can't be blamed for eating an entire frozen pizza for dinner on that day you didn't get a lunch break).

On to **carbs**—limit the refined ones, like white bread, white rice, and pastries (an occasional muffin or croissant is fine). Instead, reach for whole-grain options like whole-wheat bread, oatmeal, brown rice, barley, and popcorn (skip the butter topping). Whole grains are packed with important antioxidants, vitamins, and minerals…plus fiber (for more on which whole grains to buy, go to "The Pregnancy Pantry" on page 37). Good **protein** picks are lean cuts of meat, chicken breasts, fish (except for those on the no-no list—see "What to Shelve for Nine Months" on page 46), beans, and tofu. And stick to healthy monounsaturated **fats** and omega-3s.

How can you put all this together? For example, instead of a bowl of corn flakes, go for a combo of whole-grain cereal with fresh berries and a tablespoon of walnuts. Instead of sitting down to a huge plateful of regular spaghetti and red sauce, switch to whole-grain pasta (1 cup of cooked pasta is a serving, believe it or not) with chicken and broccoli plus sauce. Protein and fat both take longer to digest than carbohydrates, so you'll feel satisfied until your next meal. Fiber has a similar effect, and it slows the spike in blood sugar from carbohydrates. Shoot for 25 to 30 g fiber each day in your diet.

You might find that eating like this helps you lose weight. And yes, being active and staying at a healthy weight will definitely help get that body ready for mommyhood. Most women who begin their pregnancies already in shape find that it's easier to bounce back once their baby has arrived. Being **overweight** (a body mass index over 25) or **obese** (a BMI above thirty) has a negative impact on your fertility, because it impairs your ovulation. At the same time, being **underweight** will also mess with ovulation.[10] A loss or gain of only ten pounds can make all the difference for many women. Talk to your doctor or dietitian about reaching a healthy and realistic weight that's right for you.

What about **caffeine**? Well, it's definitely something you'll need to wean yourself from once you become pregnant, so you might want to save yourself the headache (literally) later, and cut back now. Numerous studies have concluded that caffeine doesn't have a significant impact on fertility, but you'll want to drop your intake to as little as possible once you're pregnant. It's a tough call whether to keep drinking your daily cuppa until you get that positive test or quit right now, so there's absolutely no risk to your unborn baby—but it could take you as long as a year to conceive. Whatever you decide, it's a smart bet to reduce the amount you're drinking to no more than a cup a day (that's the choice I made). Remember, a cup is only 8 ounces; the smallest size at Starbucks, the tall, is 12 ounces, and the venti is a honking 20 ounces. Turn to page 48 for more on caffeine and pregnancy, including a chart that lists the caffeine content of most beverages.

Soda's still okay, right? You're probably not going to like my advice: Give it up. If you're drinking the regular stuff, it's a ton of empty calories that discolor your teeth and also have a weakening effect on your bones. If you drink the diet version, you're getting artificial sweeteners, which haven't been extensively tested on pregnant women or women who are trying to get pregnant. I'm not saying that the occasional diet soda is going to hurt your chances of having a baby, but we just don't know what the long-term effects of aspartame (NutraSweet), sucralose (Splenda), and other artificial sweeteners are. I'd love to tell you that sparkling water with a twist of lime is a perfectly good substitute for your beloved cola, but you know that's just not true. If you're drinking three cans a day, try cutting back to one. And try that sparkling water: you just might like it.

Just chill. I know it's easier said than done, but **high stress levels** can sometimes affect your chances of getting pregnant due to changes in hormone levels, which can delay ovulation. In addition, not being able to get pregnant will cause you and your partner even more stress.[11] It's also true that high levels of stress during pregnancy can affect your baby. Studies show that as early as seventeen weeks into a pregnancy, the level of the stress hormone cortisol in the amniotic fluid surrounding your fetus rises at the same level as the cortisol in your blood stream. While the researchers don't know the exact effect of stress hormones on your baby, studies in animals show that high stress levels in the mother can affect brain development and behavior in offspring.[12]

Another recent study found that the babies of moms who were particularly stressed out during pregnancy had a higher risk of developing asthma and allergies. The study's authors speculate that stress may make women more susceptible to allergens, and the trait can be passed on to a fetus.[13] If you and your partner are dealing with infertility issues, you might find it useful to check out the American Fertility Association at www.afafamilymatters.com; among other resources, the organization offers weekly Internet chat sessions.

Whether it means weekly dinners with friends, regular yoga classes, escaping with trashy gossip rags (it works for me!), or making a date with your couch for *30 Rock*, make sure you relax. As long as it doesn't stress you out even more, you might want to keep a journal of how you're feeling as you launch into this next phase of life.

Sperm-Tastic

Just because you're the one with the womb, your partner's not off the hook. In fact, 50 percent of infertility is linked to the male part of the equation.[14] Encourage your hubby to get with the program and join you in your health kick, because his weight, diet, and lifestyle affect his fertility, too.

Make sure Mr. McLovin isn't smoking Cohibas and sitting in hot tubs for long periods of time (of course, you might have other reasons to question this behavior), because both smoking and exposure to high temperatures will impact his sperm quality. Those ubiquitous laptops? He shouldn't keep the computer on his lap, because the heat it generates will slow down his swimmers—and the legs-together position necessary to support the laptop doesn't help, either.[15]

A recent study of infertile men also showed that cell phone usage impacts the quality of sperm. All cell phone users were affected to some degree, but the chattiest Charlies (those who spent more than four hours talking on cell phones each day) had fewer swimmers overall, and the ones they did have were more likely to be sluggish and oddly shaped.[16] If your man is a cell phone junkie (like mine), tell him to try to keep his conversations short or use a headset.

It takes about three months for sperm to form, so urge your guy to get healthy before you plan to conceive. It might help him get with the program if you remind him that he'll need to be super-fit if he plans to keep up with the little one in your future. Oh, and mentioning what a hot dad Brad Pitt is probably wouldn't hurt with the motivation either.

Baby Daddy Diet

What's on your man's menu can affect the quality of his sperm. A recent study done by the Harvard School of Public Health found that men who ate relatively small amounts of soy daily had decreased sperm concentration, but the quality of the sperm was fine.[17] The soy industry disputed the findings, claiming that soy foods aren't linked to reduced sperm count, but my guess is that lots of women ran home and told their husbands to put the kibosh on their soy milk habit. Dr. Mark Messina, an adjunct professor at the Department of Nutrition at the School of Public Health at Loma Linda University (and pretty much the king of soy research), says that soy is fine for men and women as far as fertility goes, and adds that it's a great source of low-fat, high quality protein and B vitamins. However, he recommends eating it like the Japanese do, in the form of traditional foods rather than highly processed ones. Dr. Messina considers the optimal amount to be about two to three servings per day.

Here's what a serving of soy looks like:[18]
8-ounce glass of soy milk
½ cup tofu
⅔ cup edamame
¼ cup soy nuts
3 ounces tempeh
6 ounces soy yogurt
1 tablespoon miso

Source: Soy Foods Council

Those swimmers also need vitamin C to develop and vitamin E for movement,[19] and it turns out you're not the only one who needs folic acid. A study done at the University of California at Berkeley found that men with the highest folate intake had a 20 percent lower rate of sperm with abnormal chromosomes than men with the lowest folate intake.[20] He doesn't necessarily need to take a supplement, but make sure your guy is loading up on folic acid-rich food, just like you. I'm sure he wouldn't turn his nose up at a nice Papaya Blue Lagoon smoothie (see page 254).

A trip down the juice aisle may offer another way for your man to get super-sperm. One study (on rats, mind you) found that regular consumption of pomegranate juice can boost the quality and motility of sperm.[21] While it may be years before the same study is performed on humans, it couldn't hurt to offer your hubby a glass of pomegranate juice or a bowl of Spinach and Pear Salad with Pomegranate Dressing (see page 211). The juice of the pomegranate has significant amounts of antioxidants, which help protect all cells in the body…so why not sperm? Previous studies have confirmed pomegranate juice's potential to lower the risk of recurring prostate cancer.[22] So bottoms up!

Your Pre-Bun To-Do List

Join the Gym

Why now? Getting to a healthy weight will help improve your odds of getting pregnant. If you start an exercise program *before* you get pregnant, it'll be easier for you to maintain it during your pregnancy. That means you'll feel better, have an outlet for stress, and will probably gain less excess weight. It also might be a great way to meet other soon-to-be moms. Turn to page 103 for tips on exercise during pregnancy.

See Your Ob

It used to be that you wouldn't call your doc until you were already knocked up, but these days most ob-gyns, like Dr. Maggie R. Somerall, an obstetrician/gynecologist in Birmingham, Alabama, are encouraging their patients to schedule pre-conception visits with their partners.[23] The first prenatal visit is generally done at six to ten weeks, and a lot is going on with your baby's development by then. In order to ease your mind (and probably your spouse's, too), schedule the pre-conception visit about three months before you start trying to conceive. This allows your doctor to advise you about several topics, including current medical issues, losing or gaining weight, discontinuing any potentially harmful medication or herbal supplements, discussing family history, and getting baseline height and weight measurements. Dr. Somerall performs a complete health screening for all her obese patients to check for any underlying health issues.

Your doctor may suggest getting tested to see if you and your partner carry genes for cystic fibrosis, Tay-Sachs disease, or other inherited genetic diseases. Talk to your parents and siblings to see if any of them are carriers for hereditary diseases. You'll probably dig up some surprising information, so don't be afraid to ask. Because my husband is adopted and I'm of Eastern-European Jewish heritage, we decided to pony up for several genetic tests. Unfortunately, many insurance companies don't cover the tests, but the peace of mind you'll get from a negative test is well worth the price. And if there is an issue, it's comforting to understand your options *before* you become pregnant.

Remember when you last had a measles shot? It's probably not at the forefront of your mind, but since certain immunizations are recommended for mothers-to-be, try to find your immunization records. Your doctor will also want to know if you may be exposed to any potential environmental or occupational hazards (for example, if you work in a beauty salon or a dental practice). Your ob-gyn should ask you about your current diet and make sure you know about the importance of folic acid, and she may recommend that you begin taking prenatal vitamins. You should bring up any concerns you have and ask burning questions, such as "Can I still take my favorite spin class?" and "Can I still go on the trip we've planned to India?"

Toss Your Pills

Most ob-gyns advise that you stop taking birth control pills (or other hormone-based contraceptives) three months before trying to get preggers. It's not that it's unsafe to get pregnant immediately after going off the Pill, but it may take you a while to start ovulating normally and having regular periods—especially if you're irregular like I am. Regulating your menstrual cycle will make it easier for you to chart your cycle and therefore get pregnant. It will also help your doctor determine your date of conception. But be sure to talk to your doc; she might think addressing your "ticking clock" is more important than waiting a quarter of a year. Also, long-term use of the Pill can deplete your stores of folic acid and other B vitamins, selenium, and vitamin C, so it's smart to start a balanced diet and folate supplements before you begin trying.

See the Dentist

I know it's probably not one of your all-time faves, but it's best to see the dentist now and make sure you don't have any major dental worries. If you need X-rays or fillings, get them taken care of before you get pregnant. Researchers now know that periodontal disease (gum disease) can lead to low-birth weight and/or premature babies.

You don't need to do anything fancy—just keep up your regular good oral hygiene, brushing with fluoride toothpaste and flossing once or twice a day. Yes—flossing really does make a difference. Pregnancy hormones (hello, progesterone) and the increased blood volume that goes along with pregnancy will make your gums more swollen and inflamed, which means that if you haven't always been a flosser, you might end up with some seriously bloody gums. And oh, joy: 50 to 70 percent of all pregnant women develop gingivitis (the first stage of periodontal disease)—inflamed gums caused by plaque buildup. Even more irritating are tumors called pregnancy granulomas, which can develop on your gums due to plaque and food particles. These uncomfortable lumps (10 percent of us get them) aren't cancerous or contagious, but they can make it tough to eat and to talk. The good news? Just keep it clean, girl! A regular brushing, flossing, and rinsing routine will help prevent them.[24]

It's a good idea to see your dentist for a thorough cleaning at least once during your pregnancy, preferably during the second trimester, when it's less risky and uncomfortable for you. Of course, make sure you let her know that you've got a little bun in the oven.

Have a Girls' Weekend

…Or take a trip with the hubby. Yes, there will be time later for a babymoon, but let's face it: circumstances *will* be a bit different. There'll be no more falling into bed together for hot sex after a couple of glasses of Cabernet and salsa dancing or après-ski warmups in the hot tub. Go someplace you know will be off-limits (or at least not as much fun) later, such as Napa or South Beach. It's not likely that you're going to want to hit the bars with your friends once you're preggers (plus I don't recommend it), so live it up now, chica!

Another fun and self-indulgent move would be to take a weekend trip (or even a day trip) by yourself. Revel in a little people watching or indulge in an entire brownie in a fancy hotel bed—all by yourself. After all, once you have a little one, you won't be spending much quality time alone.

Have a "Last Supper"

Okay, remember all those things I told you to lay off on page 5? (You'll find more of them upcoming in "Chapter 5: What to Shelve for Nine Months.") Well, go ahead and eat them one more time! Go for runny cheeses, sushi, wine, and the fattest slice of chocolate cake you can find…and don't forget to finish the meal with a nice espresso.

Buy a Sexy Nightie

You'll be having sex. A lot. Probably more than you were before you were trying. Since "purposeful" sex doesn't always feel as spontaneous and steamy as when you're just fooling around for the heck of it, you might need a few fun items and outfits to help you get in the mood more often. If you and your partner haven't experimented with sex toys much or if you haven't changed your routine since your honeymoon, now's the time to get creative!

Chapter Two

Baby Bonuses and Momma Must-Haves

The Nutrients You and Your Bump Need

Most of us have a bit of an angel/devil relationship when it comes to nutrition. You have times when you're totally tuned in to what you're eating and are paying close attention to everything from calories and fat grams to how much calcium you're getting per day. But then there are moments when you're stressed, time-crunched, or blue, and you lapse into eating whatever is available, tasty, and convenient. It's completely human, and totally normal. But now that you've got a baby on board, it's time to ditch the split personality, do the right thing, and give that little guy all the tools he needs to develop.

Okay, fine, you say. *But if I wasn't taking calcium supplements or paying attention to getting enough fiber* before *I was pregnant, how can I get it together now that there are so many other things to remember?* It's natural to be nervous about getting enough of everything, but you can relax a little. First of all, your baby will snatch everything he requires and leave you with what's left, so he'll almost always get the vital nutrients he needs to grow. But if there's nothing left to run *your* overtaxed body, you'll be sluggish and more prone to getting sick. A diet that's full of variety and lots of whole foods (aka unprocessed fruits, veggies, whole grains, lean protein, and dairy) will help ensure both of you get what you need.[1]

Here's the scoop on the building blocks and how much to get of each.

Folic Acid: 600 to 800 Micrograms (mcg)

Essential to the development of your baby's spinal cord and spinal nerves, this mega-important B vitamin gets all kinds of attention; in fact, you've already heard about it in this book. It's no wonder: The vitamin plays a key role in preventing the birth defect spina bifida, and it's vital you get enough of it both before and during your pregnancy. (You also need folic acid to produce red blood cells.)

Folic acid is also one of the few vitamins that our food system is enriched with, but most women don't seem to get enough of it in their diet without supplements. If she hasn't already, your doctor will prescribe a prenatal multivitamin that contains 600 to 800 mcg of folic acid. On top of that, you'll want to pepper your diet with foods rich in folate (the natural form of the vitamin), such as oranges, asparagus, papaya, and fortified cereal. For more on getting enough folic acid before pregnancy, turn to page 1 in "Chapter 1: Trying for a Bump."

Here's a list of super-folate-rich foods:[2]

1 cup fortified cereal, like Total Raisin Bran	400 mcg
1 cup cooked lentils	358 mcg
1 cup cooked spinach	263 mcg
1 slice enriched white bread	251 mcg
1 cup edamame	200 mcg
½ cup cooked asparagus	134 mcg
2 tablespoons wheat germ	85 mcg
8 ounces orange juice	74 mcg
1 cup ripe papaya	53 mcg
1 medium orange	48 mcg

Source: nal.usda.gov

Here's another plug for getting enough folate in your diet: Low folate levels are associated with depression.[3] It's unclear whether a lack of folate causes depression, or whether depression creates low levels of this B vitamin. Either way, it's smart to eat your spinach!

Folic acid also plays a role in heart health. Folic acid, along with vitamins B_6 and B_{12}, helps break down the amino acid homocysteine in the blood; too much homocysteine can lead to atherosclerosis.[4]

Iron: 27 to 30 Milligrams

Anyone for steak? Now's the time to tuck into lean cuts of red meat, poultry, and fish. Meat is one of the major cravings during pregnancy—probably because your body is sending the message that it needs more iron. Iron is necessary for the formation of red blood cells, which your body is busy making as your blood volume increases by an incredible 50 percent. Red blood cells bring oxygen to all the muscles, tissues, and organs in your body; plus, they're in charge of bringing oxygen to your baby via the placenta. Once they've dropped off that oxygen, they pick up carbon dioxide—a waste product—and deliver it to your lungs so you can exhale it away. Since red blood cells are doing such an important job, let's make sure you have enough of them.

About half of pregnant women are iron deficient, which leads to anemia. Anemia doesn't usually have a huge effect on the health of your baby, but if it becomes severe it can lead to preterm birth and low birth weight. For you, it has the unpleasant side effect of making you feel even more tired and lackluster than you already might.[5] Your doctor will probably test you for

Belly Tip

A sprinkle a day. Adding wheat germ to the foods you eat is a really easy and tasty way to boost your folic acid intake each day. Wheat germ has a sweet, nutty flavor that's great in baked goods (just sprinkle a tablespoon or two into pancake batter or muffin mix), stirred into yogurt, or as a topping for cereal. My favorite way to use it is in a PB&J. Just shake 2 tablespoons over the peanut butter layer before you put the two slices of bread together.

anemia at your first prenatal visit and then again between twenty-four and twenty-eight weeks.[6]

You should be getting about 30 mg of iron from your prenatal vitamin, but make sure to get another 12 to 14 mg per day from your diet. As I've mentioned, iron is one of those pesky nutrients that can be difficult to absorb. To make it easier on your body, eat a vitamin C–rich food along with an iron-packed one. For more tips on that, turn to page 3.

Cooking iron-rich veggies can leach out some of their iron content, so skip boiling when it comes to your greens, and don't use a ton of water to steam vegetables like broccoli. It sounds odd, but cooking foods in a cast-iron skillet can actually boost their iron content. Cast-iron cookware is great—the only drawback is that it's heavy.

And check this out: Your little one is already hoarding enough iron to last him through the first few months of life. That's a smart move, because breast milk is low in iron (at least the form of iron in your milk is very easy for your baby to absorb), so he's stocking up on it now.[7] (Read more about breast-feeding in "Chapter 18: The Milk Factory and Beyond.") If you're a vegetarian, iron is a nutrient you need to pay extra close attention to getting. To learn more about a healthy veggie pregnancy, turn to page 75.

Belly Tip

Mighty minerals. Calcium and iron are two super-important minerals for you and your baby, but they don't get along so well. Calcium in food and supplements actually gets in the way of your body absorbing iron. You need both, so what can you do? Skip the calcium-rich foods when you eat iron-filled meals, and take calcium supplements at night before you go to bed.[8]

Pump up your diet with these easy iron sources:

Heme iron comes from an animal source; it's the easiest kind for your body to absorb.[9]

6-ounce sirloin steak	3.5 mg
3 ounces bison	3 mg

6-ounce chicken breast	2 mg
1 egg	0.6 mg
3 ounces salmon	0.5 mg

Source: nal.usda.gov

Non-heme iron: You guessed it—iron from plant-based sources. It's just as good as the kind in meat except that it's tougher for your body to absorb, so you'll need to get even more of it if you're a vegetarian.[10]

1 cup fortified cereal (Total Raisin Bran)	18 mg
1 cup cooked spinach	6.43 mg
1 cup instant fortified oatmeal	3.96 mg
1 cup cooked Swiss chard	3.95 mg
1 cup dried apricots	3.46 mg

Source: nal.usda.gov

Turn to page 75 for a long list of iron-rich vegetarian foods.

Protein: 60 Grams

It might sound like a lot, but 60 g is only about 10 more than what you needed pre-pregnancy. That extra 10 translates to roughly one protein bar, ⅓ cup of almonds, an 8-ounce yogurt, or 1½ cheese sticks. If you got on the low-carb bandwagon like everyone else did several years ago, you can probably recite all the high protein foods as easily as the names of your bridal party. The things to remember with protein are to *keep it lean* and *mix up the sources*. Most animal-based foods are good sources of protein, and legumes (including peanuts, beans of all types, and soybeans) are another rich source. Whole grains have a few grams of protein per ounce, but the real protein star in the grain world is quinoa (pronounced keen-wah).

Here are some good protein sources to include in your repertoire:[11]

3 ounces cooked beef filet	21 g
3 ounces cooked lamb	21 g
3 ounces cooked bison	24 g
3 ounces cooked pork loin	22 g
½ cooked chicken breast	29 g
3 ounces cooked turkey breast	26 g
3 ounces cooked salmon	22 g
1 large cooked egg	6 g
1 cup black beans	15 g
2 tablespoons peanut butter	8 g
1 cup cooked quinoa	8 g
8 ounces low-fat milk	8 g
5.3 ounces fat-free Greek yogurt	13 g
1 cup edamame	17 g

Source: nal.usda.gov and National Turkey Federation

Choline: 450 Milligrams

Heard of choline? Probably not. This nutrient doesn't get much play in the media, but it's essential for your baby's brain development and prevention of birth defects. It may even help your child's memory and ability to learn down the road, because choline plays a role in the development of the hippocampus, which is the memory center of the brain.[12] Pregnant women need 450 mg of choline per day, and if you breast-feed, that requirement jumps to 550 mg.[13]

Where do you get it? The sources are pretty slim—only chicken liver, beef liver, eggs, wheat germ, and cauliflower offer substantial amounts. Obviously, eggs are the most convenient and versatile source, and they offer plenty—250 mg in two eggs. But don't ditch that yolk—that's where choline and plenty of other amazing nutrients are. And by the way, the cholesterol in egg yolks does not raise your blood cholesterol levels, and the American Heart Association says it's fine to eat one egg per day.

Here's a breakdown of the other choline-rich foods:[14]

¼ cup wheat germ	50 mg

(See Belly Tip on page 17 for adding wheat germ to your diet.)

½ cup dry roasted soybeans	107 mg
1 cup cooked cauliflower	48 mg
4-ounce pork chop	95 mg

Source: nal.usda.gov

And the news on choline just keeps getting better. New research out of the National Institutes of Health (NIH) found that women with high choline intake had a 24 percent lower risk of developing breast cancer. Of the 3,000 study participants, the women with the highest choline intake received about 455 mg or more, while the lowest consumed 195 mg or less per day.[15]

Evidently, only 10 percent of Americans are getting enough of this essential nutrient. In addition to its baby benefits and apparent breast-cancer protection, choline also plays a role in heart health by helping to reduce homocysteine (just like folic acid).

Get your hands on choline with these recipes:

Huevos Rancheros Wrap (page 237)

Everything but the Kitchen Sink Frittata (page 204)

Chunky Monkey Muffins (page 158)

Calcium: 1,000 Milligrams

Yep—it's the same amount you needed before pregnancy (unless you're a teenager). But if you don't live on a dairy farm, you're probably not getting that much each day. Most women only get 750 mg a day, so it's time to bone up.[16] In addition to keeping *your* bones and teeth strong, calcium is also required to get Junior's structure off to a solid start. Even though your calcium requirement doesn't increase, pregnancy makes it much more important to actually get that whole 1,000 mg. If you don't supply calcium through your diet, Baby will get creative and start pulling it from your bones (yikes!).

Dairy is a great source of calcium, but you can also find it in everything from beans to broccoli (see chart on page 77 in vegetarian section).

Here are the top ten sources of calcium:[17]

8 ounces plain yogurt	415 mg
3 ounces sardines with bones	324 mg
1½ ounces cheddar cheese	306 mg
8 ounces skim milk	302 mg
8 ounces 2% milk	297 mg
1½ ounces part-skim mozzarella	275 mg
6 ounces calcium-fortified orange juice	263 mg
3 ounces canned salmon (with bones)	181 mg
½ cup chocolate pudding made with 2% milk	153 mg
1 cup 1% cottage cheese	138 mg
½ cup tofu made with calcium sulfate	138 mg

Source: nal.usda.gov

To help you get more calcium, I've boosted the bone-building factor in many of the recipes in this book by adding dry milk powder to the recipe. It might sound a little weird, but it's an easy way to get a nutrient boost without changing the flavor. You can try it in smoothies, soups, and other tasty items like muffins and quickbreads.

Try these calcium-rich recipes, which offer at least 10 percent of your daily requirement:

Better Than Elvis Milkshake (page 157)

Brocco Mac and Cheese (page 222)

Citrus-Spiked Rice Pudding (page 165)

Vitamin D: 200 to 400 International Units (IU)

Vitamin D is the trusty sidekick that helps calcium and phosphorus get absorbed by the body. In recent years, vitamin D has been touted as the next super nutrient; it's been linked to preventing cancer, boosting the immune system, and reducing inflammation. It also helps increase muscle strength, which couldn't hurt right now.

You need the same amount as you did before your pregnancy, but now it's super-vital that you get enough. (Several experts are now advocating 1000 IU of Vitamin D each day for everyone.) You can get it from food (see the chart on the following page), but your skin can also make its own vitamin D with direct exposure to the sun. For those in sunny climes, that's easy, but mommas stuck up north may need to make an extra effort to catch some rays in the winter. Plus, now that we've all finally started wearing sunscreen religiously, we're blocking our ability to make vitamin D naturally right along with those harmful UV rays. In addition, pollution (hello, ladies in L.A., Pittsburgh, and Houston[18]) blocks your skin's ability to make the vitamin, as does having darker skin. Ask your doctor whether she suggests taking a supplement.

Just fifteen minutes a day of direct sunlight is enough for your skin to make vitamin D[19]…a great excuse to bask in those sweet rays without feeling guilty. Just make sure to cover up after that golden fifteen.

Most vitamin D-rich foods come from the sea. The richest source is from—gag—cod liver oil. If you can choke it down, more power to you!

Dig into these more palatable vitamin D-rich foods:[20]

3½ ounces salmon	360 IUs
3½ ounces mackerel	345 IUs
1¾ ounces sardines	250 IUs
3 ounces tuna fish	200 IUs
1 cup milk (all types) fortified with vitamin D	98 IUs
1 cup fortified cereal (like Total)	40 IUs
1 egg	20 IUs

Source: nal.usda.gov

Omega-3 (in the Form of DHA): 200 Milligrams

Turn to "Chapter 7: Go Fish" for more on this essential nutrient.

Fiber: 28 to 30 Grams

If you have friends who have already been through a pregnancy, they've probably clued you in to the fact that they got a little, uh, backed up during those nine months. Most women don't get enough fiber to begin with, and pregnancy increases the requirement by about 12 percent, which means 28 to 30 g a day. Lots of things can make you constipated when you're pregnant: slowed digestion, dehydration, dietary changes, iron supplements, and decreased activity. Here's the trick—get a jump start on your fiber intake each morning with whole-grain cereal: Some have as much as 10 g of fiber per serving. Then, fit more in at each meal and snack; it's easy if you're eating plenty of fruits, veggies, and grains. Remember: The more fiber you eat, the more water you need to drink to keep everything flowing.

Keep things moving with these fiber-rich foods:[21]

1 ounce almonds	17 g
1 cup cooked black beans	15 g
1 cup Kashi GoLean cereal	10 g
1 large pear	7 g
1 cup cooked whole-wheat pasta	6 g
1 Kellogg's All-Bran Bar	5 g
1 slice Wasa crisp bread	2 g

Source: nal.usda.gov

Fiber-rich recipes to keep things moving (at least 3 g of fiber per serving):

Chunky Monkey Muffins (page 158)

Pregnancy Pad Thai (page 241)

Fresh Fruit with Creamy Yo-Co Dip (page 175)

Belly Tip

Fiber will be your friend post-pregnancy, too. Since it helps you feel full longer, it's an important tool for weight loss.

B Vitamins (B_6, B_{12}, Thiamin, and Riboflavin)

Vitamin B_{12} is one of those miracle vitamins. It helps keep your nerve cells and red blood cells healthy, and it's also vital for making your DNA. During pregnancy, you need to get 2.6 mcg a day. B_{12} is also a component of breast milk, so if you're not getting enough, your baby won't get enough. Since

B_{12} is supplied by animal-derived foods like poultry, fish, meat, eggs, and dairy, moms who follow vegetarian or vegan diets may be deficient.[22] B_{12} is important for your baby's neurologic development, so talk to your pediatrician about using a B_{12} supplement if you don't get any animal products in your diet.[23]

Luckily, not all the B vitamins are so tough to find. B_6 is found in lots of everyday foods like baked potatoes (with skin), fortified cereal, instant oatmeal, garbanzo beans, and bananas. B_6 is important for metabolism of protein and red blood cells, and you need it to make hemoglobin, the component of red blood cells that carries oxygen to your body's tissues. In fact, like not getting enough iron, a B_6 deficiency can also cause anemia. B_6 is vital for your immune system to function properly, which is super important when you're pregnant. During pregnancy, you need 1.9 mg a day, but it's pretty easy to meet your needs as long as you eat a variety of foods.[24]

Here's yet another reason to eat your whole grains. They're rich in thiamin, aka vitamin B_1, which is important for carbohydrate metabolism and nerve conduction. It's found in pork, beans, and whole grains, such as brown rice. Pregnancy and breast-feeding both increase requirements to 1.4 mg a day. Thiamin deficiency has been linked to hyperemesis gravidarum, which is a severe form of pregnancy-related nausea and vomiting (turn to page 87 for more on that).[24] Finally, there's vitamin B_2, which is known as riboflavin. You'll find it in those ever-popular organ meats, milk, bread, and fortified cereals. Your needs during pregnancy increase slightly to 1.4 mg a day, and they go up a bit higher if you're breast-feeding. Your prenatal vitamin should have a good supply of both thiamin and riboflavin.[25]

Here are some great ways to get your Bs:

B_{12} (2.6 mcg/day)[26]

3 ounces salmon	2.6 mcg
¼ pound hamburger	2.2 mcg
8 ounces of 1% milk	1 mcg

B$_6$ (1.9 mg/day)[27]

¾ cup Total whole-grain cereal	2 mg
1 small baked potato with skin	0.47 mg
1 cup fortified instant oatmeal (such as Quaker Original)	0.45 mg
1 banana	0.43 mg
1 cup brown rice	0.28 mg

B$_1$ (thiamin; 1.4 mg/day)[28]

¾ cup Total whole-grain cereal	1.5 mg
1 pork chop	0.7 mg
1 cup garbanzo beans	0.26 mg

B$_2$ (riboflavin; 1.4 mg/day)[29]

¾ cup Total whole-grain cereal	1.7 mg
8 ounces chocolate milk	0.42 mg
1 plain Thomas' English muffin	0.16 mg

Source: nal.usda.gov

Iodine: 220 Micrograms

Something tells me this mineral hasn't really crossed your mind much. Iodine has been added to our table salt since the 1920s, but studies show that its iodine content may be less than what the label shows. Plus, these days many people use fancy sea salts and kosher salt in their cooking, and since those salts aren't iodized, you may not be getting enough. The number of women with iodine deficiency has risen in the last thirty years. Iodine is necessary for thyroid hormone production and for preventing goiter, which is an enlarged thyroid gland.

When you're pregnant, your need for iodine increases by a hefty 70 mcg a day, to 220 mcg.[30] Iodine deficiency can put your baby at risk for impaired physical and mental development. Women with autoimmune diseases like lupus are more prone to having low levels of iodine.[31]

There's no need to salt up your food, but use iodized salt in your everyday cooking (save the fancy stuff for company). Also, make sure your prenatal vitamin contains iodine.

Other good sources of iodine are milk, seaweed (sushi's out, but order an avocado-and-cucumber roll), seafood, and eggs, plus:[32]

1 teaspoon iodized salt	400 mcg
3 ounces haddock	125 mcg
½ cup cottage cheese	49 mcg
3 ounces shrimp	29 mcg

*Source: Northwestern University Feinberg
School of Nutrition Fact Sheet on Iodine*

Niacin and Pantothenic Acid

These are other micronutrients that you really don't need to think about on a daily basis because our food supply is loaded with them. They might be a little familiar because you've seen them on the side of your fortified cereal box. Yes, cereal is a good source of both of these vitamins. Other whole grains, plus meat, fish, and poultry are great sources, too. The pantothenic acid requirement during pregnancy is 6 mg per day, and niacin's is 18 mg per day.[33]

Try these foods:[34]

1 cooked pork chop	12 mg niacin, 0.84 mg pantothenic acid
1 cup cooked brown rice	3 mg niacin, 0.6 mg pantothenic acid

3 ounces halibut	6 mg niacin, 0.32 mg pantothenic acid
1 cup cooked chicken	18 mg niacin, 1.3 mg pantothenic acid

Source: nal.usda.gov

Vitamin C: 85 Milligrams

This powerful antioxidant is in everything these days from throat drops to facial moisturizer. That's because vitamin C has the power to fight free radicals and the oxidative damage they cause to your cells. In plain English, that means that free radicals do what your husband (okay, my husband) does when he comes into a room: gets crumbs on the couch, puts his shoes up on the ottoman, and generally leaves things a bit ruffed up. Just like you, vitamin C swoops in and brings back order.

Your pregnant body needs 85 mg of vitamin C each day, and that's pretty easy to get via fruits, vegetables, and fruit juices.[35] One of the most common cravings during pregnancy is for fruit—especially citrus—and the increased need for vitamin C and folate may be what's behind that.

Top sources of vitamin C:[36]

1 cup raw bell pepper	118 mg
1 cup cooked Brussels sprouts	97 mg
1 cup strawberries	89 mg
1 cup fresh papaya	87 mg
1 cup raw broccoli	81 mg
1 medium kiwifruit	71 mg
1 medium orange	64 mg
1 cup fresh cantaloupe	59 mg

6 ounces tomato juice	50 mg
½ pink grapefruit	46 mg
1 cup raw cauliflower	46 mg
1 cup cherry tomatoes	19 mg

Source: nal.usda.gov

Vitamin A: 770 Micrograms (About 2,565 International Units [IU]*)

This fat-soluble vitamin plays a starring role in baby's development. It's vital for skin and eye cell growth, and it's necessary for a healthy immune system. The trick with vitamin A is that while it's very important to get enough during pregnancy, it's also possible to get too much. Large amounts of vitamin A are actually teratogenic, which means that they can cause birth defects. The amount of vitamin A that you get from your diet and your prenatal multivitamin *combined* shouldn't be more than 3,000 mcg (10,000 IU) of vitamin A per day.[37]

So what gives? How do you get enough without overdoing it? Vitamin A is plentiful in the food supply. You'll find it in animal products, fortified dairy products, fish, and dark-colored fruits and veggies. Plus, it'll likely be in your prenatal vitamin (take a look—some have as much as 4,000 IU), so make sure not to double up on those.

Vitamin A comes in two forms, like iron: preformed vitamin A and beta-carotene. The preformed variety is found in animal-derived products, including beef and chicken livers and dairy products, as well as supplements.[38] That's the kind that you don't want to go overboard on. The one food I would advise against is liver (especially beef), because it can have as much as 28,000 IU per 3-ounce serving. If you absolutely crave it, avoid it during the first trimester and limit your overall consumption to no more than once a month.

Beta-carotene is found in plant food sources, including carrots, spinach, kale, cantaloupe, papaya, sweet potatoes, mangoes, and apricots—basically

---

* Most vitamins aren't measured in IU, but vitamins A and D often show up as IU.

anything with an orange or dark green tint. That form is perfectly safe, even in large quantities. The most it will do is turn your skin orange.

Magnesium: 350 to 360 Milligrams

Along with calcium and vitamin D, the mineral magnesium is part of the bone-building team. During pregnancy, you need between 350 and 360 mg per day, depending on your age. Foods that are rich in magnesium (over 100 mg per serving) include spinach, pumpkin seeds, Brazil nuts, and black beans.[39]

Good sources include:[40]

¼ cup roasted pumpkin seeds	303 mg
1 cup cooked spinach	157 mg
1 cup black beans	120 mg
1 ounce (6 pieces) Brazil nuts	107 mg
3 ounces halibut	91 mg

Source: nal.usda.gov

Zinc: 11 Milligrams

This mineral helps keep your immune system kicking and regulates gene expression, the process in which a gene is switched on in a cell to make RNA and proteins. If you're a vegetarian, you can't absorb zinc from food as well, so make sure to up your intake of zinc-rich foods.[41]

Fortified cereals, red meat, and seafood are all good sources; below are some specifics:[42]

1 cup Total raisin bran	15 mg
3 ounces sirloin steak	6 mg
3-ounce pork chop	2.9 mg

8 ounces plain yogurt	2 mg
3 ounces shrimp	1.3 mg

Source: nal.usda.gov

Fluids

The Institute of Medicine recommends that pregnant women drink 10 cups (2.4 liters) of water each day. It's smart to get in the habit now, because if you decide to breast-feed, that requirement increases to 12.5 cups (3 liters) each day. That's a whole lot—not to mention the fact that you're already running to the bathroom like it's your part-time job—but you need it, because your blood volume (the amount of blood in your body) is on the rise. Dehydration can make your nausea worse, and it can cause contractions in your second and third trimester.

But all this liquid doesn't have to only come from plain water. You can drink milk, soy milk, lemonade, watered-down juice, decaf iced tea, and so on. Turn to page 249 in the recipe chapter for lots of tasty, not-overly-sugary options.

Belly Tip

Drinking buddy. Here's a tip for getting yourself to drink more water. Buy a pretty glass and keep it at your desk. Seriously—it works! If you have something that you actually *want* to drink out of, you're more likely to do it. And if you work at home or have a fridge at work, fill up a pitcher of water (most hold about 2 to 2.5 quarts) and keep refilling your glass all day. If you can't do that, hopefully your workplace has a watercooler. You'll just have to get up and refill more often, but since you're peeing pretty much every forty-five minutes, you have a good reason to get up anyway.

Calories: 300 Extra a Day—Yay!

Yes, you'll need more energy to burn, but you're not eating for two and your body doesn't require the extra 300 until your second trimester.[43] This is one thing that you won't have a tough time getting. It's incredibly easy to add 300 calories to your daily diet. The tough thing is to get them from healthy, baby-building calories, instead of caramel-drizzled brownie calories, but that's where my Momma Munchies (see page 140) come in handy. If you're starting out your pregnancy already over- or underweight, your doctor should help you customize your recommended extra calories.

Chapter Three

She's Gotta Have It

Why You Crave What You Crave, And How to Deal with It

As I hinted earlier, researchers still don't know why pregnancy brings on all sorts of food cravings and aversions; the science is inconclusive. Some think that food cravings are simply learned behaviors: If society tells you you're going to crave things while you're pregnant, you will. But other researchers feel strongly that we crave foods that are rich in the nutrients we need for a healthy pregnancy. Since not all women experience cravings during pregnancy (about 85 percent of us do), it's tough to come to any conclusions about whether they serve a purpose.[1]

Now what about all the stuff that's making your stomach turn? Is there a reason behind it? Food aversions are also common in pregnancy, which is why you might not be able to deal with handling raw chicken or beef anymore, and why the smell of freshly brewed coffee has suddenly switched from your favorite morning scent to a stomach-turning stench. Again, science can't support *or* refute whether these aversions have anything to do with keeping you and your growing baby safe. Common sense might tell you that your body is trying to keep you away from anything that might hurt your baby, such as caffeine. But then again, some women find themselves totally turned off by green vegetables during pregnancy. So go figure.

You might think the foods you're craving are weird, or at least out of the norm for you. In fact, your likes and dislikes can definitely change during pregnancy. A friend of mine who is completely lactose intolerant couldn't get enough dairy while she was pregnant, and it didn't cause her the usual digestive grief. It was all she could do to not throw a fit when her work cafeteria didn't have chocolate pudding. Indeed, dairy products (including ice cream and cheese) are a common pregnancy craving. Other biggies include sweets, chocolate, fruits (especially citrus), and fish.[2]

Sometimes your taste preferences will change for good. My friend Maria had a huge sweet tooth before she had her son. During her pregnancy, she completely lost her taste for cookies, cakes, and the like, and developed a craving for Mediterranean foods instead. She's still eating lots of hummus and olives, and never regained her love of sweets.

And it turns out that women with more cravings also have more aversions. So even though you're cutting certain foods out of your diet, you may be making up for them nutritionally with other foods that you now can't get enough of.[3]

That schnoz of yours has become hyper-alert, causing things to smell odd or stronger than usual. Studies have shown that pregnant women have increased sensitivity to smells.[4] Your new bloodhound abilities may make you more prone to food aversions, nausea, and vomiting. The Chanel No. 5 that used to be your signature scent may now seem incredibly overwhelming, and stepping into your favorite deli might leave you running for fresh air. While these olfactory offenses may be annoying to you, they might also be a way of making sure you stay away from potentially harmful things. My mother found that the scent of coffee made her queasy, so she really didn't have much trouble giving it up during pregnancy.

Even if you haven't yet experienced food cravings firsthand, you've probably had friends regale you with stories of their 7 a.m. drive-through burgers, or afternoon snacks of an entire box of Entenmann's cake donuts. Whatever weird cravings or repulsions you do develop, don't get too hung up on them. As long as you're making an effort to eat a wide variety of healthy, unprocessed foods, you'll most likely be getting what you need. Plus, those queasies should calm down after the first trimester, so just eat as much of the healthy stuff as you can muster and make sure to take your prenatal vitamins.

What if you're craving paint chips instead of potato chips? You may have pica. Pica is a condition where pregnant women crave nonfood items, such as dirt, paint chips, soap, clay, laundry starch, corn starch, or ashes. Not only can these things make you sick to your stomach, they can be downright dangerous. If you crave any of the items above—or anything else that isn't food related—call your doctor immediately.[5] Some experts say pica may be a sign of severe nutritional deficiencies in iron and calcium, so there's yet another reason to keep eating right.

Belly Tip

Go halfsies. Jonesing for a strawberry milkshake or a thick slice of carrot cake? Go for it, but since these foods are sugary and rich (and often come in super-size portions), split them with someone else. If you don't have someone there to eat half when the craving strikes, ask your server before the food arrives to cut the portion in half and box the rest up, or ask her to just bring you half a serving. It sounds kind of silly, but most places are more than happy to accommodate you. You'd be surprised how much pull a pregnant woman has.

Chapter Four

The Pregnancy Pantry

A well-stocked pantry makes putting a meal on the table so much easier—now more than ever before. You don't have the time or the energy to waste rummaging around for good-for-you ingredients to feed your belly. I've put together this overview of a pregnancy pantry so that trip to the store is a little easier.

Ideally, you'll always have essentials, like whole-grain cereals, organic milk, extra-virgin olive oil, and walnuts at the ready, and you'll just need a few additional fresh items to whip up the recipes at the end of the book. I find it easiest to do a big shopping trip once a week, and then fill in once or twice a week with a few recipe-specific items. Keep a running shopping list on your fridge, and when you run out of something, add it to the list.

You don't need to dash to the health-food store and load up your cart; most of the foods I'm recommending can be found at your regular grocery store. But there are certain specialty items you'll need to make the recipes in this book (flax seeds, wheat germ, omega-3 enhanced eggs, etc.), as well as a few kitchen tools that will make your life easier.

We've all heard that we should stick to the perimeter of the grocery store (fresh produce, dairy case) and steer clear of the center aisles (processed and packaged foods) as much as possible. While this is true to some extent, there's a whole lot of good stuff happening in the frozen section and the cereal and nut aisles. In fact, studies have shown that flash freezing (which is how all modern day frozen fruits and veggies are prepared) seals in polyphenols in produce.[1] Flash freezing also means that individual pieces of fruit or vegetables are frozen, yielding firm results instead of a mushy clod. On the other hand, fresh produce that treks from California to your New Jersey grocery store and then sits there for three days before you bring it home may lose significant amounts of disease-fighting phytonutrients (antioxidants) due to damage from light and heat.

One more thing to consider: Sometimes it's good to be dense—as in nutrient-dense, which means that calorie for calorie, a food contains high amounts of nutrients. For example, if you compared 100 calories of potato chips to 100 calories of avocado, the avocado would provide substantial amounts of folate, potassium, monounsaturated fats, and fiber, and the potato chips would give you mostly fat and empty calories. You could do the same comparison between a regular chocolate-chip cookie and one made with whole-grain flour and cranberries. See what I mean? It's like spending $100 on an amazing pair of Jimmy Choos that are on a mega sale instead of paying $100 for a mediocre pair of shoes: You're spending the same amount, but you're getting a lot more bang for your buck. As much as possible, I'll steer you toward the densest food choices so you max out your calories for the day.

SHOPPING LIST

Here's a reproducible shopping list to stock up your pregnancy pantry. You can tear it out and make copies, or download it at my website: www.franceslargemanroth.com.

Produce

- Bagged, ready-to-eat, **spinach**.

- **Broccoli** (winter), **asparagus** (spring), **snap peas** (summer), and **Brussels sprouts** (fall).

- Organic **cherry tomatoes**.

- **Oranges, grapefruit,** and **tangerines** (winter); **peaches, plums,** and **nectarines** (spring); **berries** and **melon** (summer); and **apples, pears,** and **grapes** (fall).

- **Carrots** (baby or regular).

Refrigerated Section

- **Orange** or **grapefruit juice**.

- **Pomegranate juice**.

- **Hummus** or **baba ghanoush**.

Dairy

- **Organic cottage cheese** (Nancy's is a good brand).

- **Organic 1% milk** or **soy milk**.

- **Organic string cheese** and **shredded cheese**.

- Low-fat cups of **organic yogurt** (Wallaby and Stonyfield Farm are great brands).

- **Organic kefir** (a yogurty drink that's rich in probiotics).

Cereal and Bread

- **Enriched whole-grain cereal**, like Total.

- Other **whole-grain cereal** with at least 4 g fiber per serving.

- **Whole-grain tortillas** or **wraps**.

- **Whole-wheat English muffins**.

- **Rolled oats** (the old-fashioned kind).

- Low-sugar **instant fortified oatmeal** (go for a plain variety or one with less than 20 g of sugar per serving; Nature's Path is a good one to try).

- **Whole-grain, reduced-sodium crackers** (Kashi is a good pick).

- **Wheat germ**.

Pasta, Grains, and Nuts

- **Whole-wheat pasta**. If you're not a big fan of the really grainy stuff, go for a multi-grain one, like Barilla Plus.

- **Quinoa**. This tough-to-pronounce (keen-wa) ancient grain is quick cooking and packed with calcium and protein, making it a must-have for vegetarian moms-to-be.

- **Whole, unsalted almonds**. Fiber- and calcium-rich and tasty to boot, these nuts are perfect for snacking or adding to cereal or

The Pregnancy Pantry   41

salads. Package them in snack-size ziplock bags, and keep them in your purse, desk, glove compartment, or diaper bag.

- **Whole walnuts.** Super-rich tasting and a good source of vegetarian omega-3s, walnuts are a pantry star. Chop and add to oatmeal and spinach salads, or add to cookies, such as the Oh, Baby! Breakfast Cookies on page 183.

- **Natural peanut butter and almond butter** (with no hydrogenated oil or high-fructose corn syrup).★ This was probably relegated to post-workout snack food before you were pregnant. Now, with its substantial amounts of quick protein, it'll be your best friend. Use it to make PB&Js, of course, but also try PB&Bs (bananas) or PB&As (crunchy apple slices). Jars are great when you're at home, but for travel and office snacking, try Justin's Nut Butters (www.justinsnutbutter.com), which come in various fabulous flavors and are packaged in neat foil 200-calorie-or-less packs, which fit perfectly into your purse.

Meat/Poultry/Eggs/Soy Protein

- **Organic omega-3 DHA-enhanced eggs**. These eggs are from chickens that have been fed a vegetarian diet rich in microalgae. Gold Circle is a good brand to try, with 150 mg of DHA per egg.

- **Natural or organic boneless, skinless chicken breasts** and/or **cutlets**.

★*A word on allergies. Researchers have not been able to conclusively link a mother's PB consumption with allergies in her child. But some studies suggest that pregnant women who consumed nut products daily increased their child's risk of asthma by 50 percent. Moderate amounts of peanuts and peanut butter haven't been found to produce the same effect. If peanut allergy runs in your family, talk to your doctor before making the nutty spread a regular snack.[2]*

- **Salmon fillets** (ask the fishmonger to remove the skin for you). Wild salmon is healthier than farmed, but there's been a global shortage of wild salmon for the past few years, and if you can find it, it may cost up to $20 a pound.

- **Tofu**. I like extra-firm tofu for stir-fries because it actually stays together when you cook it. For increasing the protein in smoothies, soups, or dips, try soft or silken tofu. Marinated ready-to-eat tofu steaks are a super invention, too: Just make sure to check the sodium and choose one with less than 500 mg per serving.

Frozen

- **Any type of berries**. Packed with antioxidants and fiber, frozen berries are a must-have when fresh berries are out of season. Throw them into smoothies, muffins, and hot cereal.

- **Edamame**, whole or shelled.

- **Mixed veggies**. The more colors you can find, the better.

- **Brown rice**. This super time-saver is a godsend. Instead of spending forty-five minutes (or about fifteen for Minute Rice) making the whole-grain variety, just pop already-cooked frozen brown rice into the microwave for a few minutes and it's ready. Of course, if you prefer making it from scratch, that's great too.

- **Ice cream**. Go for regular if you're only indulging once in a while, but if this is your new vice, go for one of the good reduced-fat, slow-churned brands like Edy's. Unfortunately, I haven't been able to find a really good light organic ice cream that's available nationwide.

- **Shrimp**. You can get these already peeled, deveined, and cooked, which means all you need to do is defrost and add them to pasta (see page 203) or rice or wrap them up in a tortilla with some salsa. You can also ask your fishmonger to steam fresh ones.

Staples

- **Extra-virgin olive oil**. Olive oil is good, but virgin and extra-virgin olive oils are even better. Basically, extra virgin is the first press of the olive to extract the oil, which means that all the goodies from the olives, like phenols, are still intact. Regular olive oil is produced from several pressings of the olive, and it's lower in health-promoting properties. Store your olive oil away from light and heat, which is kind of tough in a kitchen, right? Keep it in either a tinted glass bottle or a metal container. If you buy oil in a super-large bottle or tin, transfer it to a smaller bottle or can that you can use for everyday, and store the rest away in a cool place to keep it fresh. I primarily use olive oil in my recipes, not only because I love the flavor, but also because it's a healthy fat. Extra-virgin olive oil has also been shown to help reduce blood clotting factors, which is particularly important during and after pregnancy, when you're more susceptible to dangerous blood clots.

- **Balsamic vinegar**. This aged vinegar is great for whipping up homemade dressings, marinating meat and tofu, and even drizzling on strawberries. For many women, it's one of the few remedies that helps quell nausea.

- **Pure cranberry juice**. This is 100 percent cranberry juice, not to be confused with cranberry juice cocktail; it's so tart that it's barely drinkable on its own. But it's great for mixing with other juices or plain sparkling water. You'll find it in the non-refrigerated juice aisle.

Must-Have Gadgets

- A **three-in-one pot** with both draining and steamer baskets (perfect for making pasta and steaming veggies at the same time).

- A **large (10 to 12-inch) sauté or frying pan**.

- One or two **baking sheets**.

- A **Microplane grater** is excellent for grabbing the zest of citrus fruit without getting any of its bitter white pith. Zest is great for adding flavor to foods without adding any fat.

- Two (or more) **plastic or ceramic cutting boards**.

- **Kitchen shears** let you chop herbs without bruising them. They're also helpful for trimming the fat from chicken or cutting spaghetti in half.

- **Chef's knife**. For tips on handling knives, turn to page 138 in "Chapter 15: Belly in the Kitchen."

- **Paring knife**.

- **Colander**.

- **Citrus juicer** or reamer for fresh lemon or lime juice.

- A few **silicone spatulas**.

- **Blender**.

- Some type of **food processor**.

- **Hand or stand mixer**.

Nice to Have

- **Two Silpat mats** for baking and toasting nuts.

- **Grill pan**.

- **Toaster oven** that can toast *and* bake, thus saving you from bending over and lifting when you only have small items to bake.

Chapter Five

What to Shelve for Nine Months

Here it comes—that long list of things that you have to kick to the curb while you're pregnant. It might cramp your style for a while, but it's well worth it. Some women find they can't remember all the foods on the no-no list, so there's a cheat sheet on page xxi. Make a copy for your purse so you'll always be able to refer to it—even on the sly.

Tobacco

I know it goes without saying that if you're smart enough to be reading this book right now, you're smart enough to know that it's incredibly damaging to smoke while you're pregnant. That said, according to the March of Dimes, 10 percent of pregnant women in the United States still smoke during their pregnancies. So here it is one more time—don't do it.

Smoking during pregnancy doubles your risk of having a low-birth weight baby (a baby weighing less than 5½ pounds at birth) because it slows fetal growth. Smoking has also been shown to increase the risk of preterm delivery (birth before thirty-seven weeks).[1] Smoking can also cause issues with the placenta, such as placenta previa (obstruction of the cervix by the placenta) and placental abruption (detachment of the placenta from the uterus before or during labor).[2]

Once the baby of a mom who smokes is born, the news gets even worse. These babies are born addicted to nicotine and are more difficult to soothe.

Plus, their risk of dying from Sudden Infant Death Syndrome (SIDS) is three times higher than babies of moms who didn't smoke.[3]

Secondhand smoke is no joke either. If you are regularly exposed to secondhand smoke (either from a family member or in your work environment), your baby's growth may be slowed and she may have a low birth weight, which can result in other complications.[4] Try to avoid smoky environments as much as possible. Thankfully, most states have banned smoking in public places, like restaurants and bars. The glaring exceptions? Alabama, Michigan, New Hampshire, North Carolina (no big surprise, since it's the largest tobacco-growing state), South Carolina, and Virginia. Let's hope they hurry up and get with the program![5]

Alcohol

I know what you're thinking: *Of course* you're not planning to drink like a fish while you're pregnant, but an occasional sip won't hurt, right? The French and Italian drink wine when they're pregnant, and they seem fine. Well, today even the French and the Brits—who've historically advocated a good pint of Guinness for a healthy pregnancy—have now started to warn their citizens about the effects of alcohol during pregnancy. And well they should. Each year, forty thousand babies in this country suffer the adverse effects of alcohol.[6]

Fetal alcohol spectrum disorder includes various types of birth defects, such as mental retardation, learning and behavioral disabilities, and others. The most severe is fetal alcohol syndrome, which is a combination of both mental and physical defects.[7]

According to the March of Dimes, there is no safe level of alcohol during pregnancy, so better safe than sorry. Because alcohol passes directly from the mother to the fetus through the placenta, there's no way to protect your baby from absorbing the booze. Before you freak out about that mojito you drank the night you conceived or the bottle of wine you shared with your best friend when you were a few weeks pregnant and didn't know it, relax. It happens to a lot of women. The important thing is that you stop drinking once you've gotten that positive pregnancy test.

So fine, you're not going to touch a drop of the stuff while you're preg-gers. You know to avoid glasses of prosecco and shots of tequila, but alcohol also sneaks up in some less obvious places. Around the holidays, many cakes are soaked in bourbon, and sweets like (my family's fave) rum balls abound. If people put treats out at the office, or if there's something at a party that you're not sure about, subtly ask the host what's in her divine creation. You could also just give it a discreet sniff—the fumes are usually a dead giveaway.

What about cooking? Doesn't all the alcohol burn off? That's what I thought, but unfortunately, it's not always true. A baked good that has been cooked for an hour still contains 25 percent of its original alcohol levels. Foods that are marinated in a mixture that contains alcohol and then grilled will retain quite a bit of residual alcohol. A dish like pasta with vodka sauce contains about 40 percent of its original alcohol level.[8] Ask whenever you're in doubt. If someone gets annoyed that you're being persnickety, give him your sincerest smile and tell him you're just trying to do right by your baby.

Obviously, the decision about whether to imbibe occasionally is a very personal one that's based on your upbringing and cultural traditions. I have several friends who told me they enjoyed small glasses of wine on occasion during their pregnancies. Some doctors say it's okay to kick back with a glass of wine or beer once the baby is fully developed and ready to arrive in a matter of days or hours. Of course, always make sure to check with your doctor before popping the cork.

Caffeine (for the Most Part)

Most expert recommendations have allowed up to 300 mg of caffeine a day for pregnant women. But a January 2008 study from the Kaiser Permanente Division of Research showed a strong link between caffeine consumption—whether from coffee, soda, tea, energy drinks, or hot chocolate—and miscar-riage. The study followed women who did not change their caffeine intake during pregnancy. The women who consumed 200 mg of caffeine a day had double the risk of miscarrying than women who didn't have any. And women who consumed less than 200 mg were 40 percent more likely to miscarry than women who had no caffeine.[9]

What does 200 mg look like? About two 8-ounce cups of regular drip coffee or about four 8-ounce cups of black tea, or about two and a half Red Bulls. The risk seems to be from the caffeine itself, not other compounds in these drinks.

I realize that this is not only scary, but also a major bummer—especially during that first trimester when you scarcely have the energy to drag your carcass up a flight of stairs. But there are other means besides caffeine to feel energized. Here's a short list:

- **Take a walk**. A brisk, ten-minute walk outside can give you Kelly Ripa perkiness. Okay, maybe not quite, but it *can* help clear the cobwebs.

- **Do some energizing stretches**. Reach your arms out to your sides and up over your head while you breathe in deeply. Exhale as you slowly lower your arms. Deep inhalations through your nose, followed by slow exhalations out through your mouth, can help you feel more alert. Turn to page 107 in "Chapter 12: Sweating for Two" for a series of energizing and restorative yoga poses.

- **Hydrate**. Drink a glass of sparkling water with a spritz of lemon juice. Dehydration can also make you feel tired.

- **Take a sniff**. Naturopathic medicine and aromatherapy practitioners tout that scents can alter your mood. It may not work for you, but it's worth a try. According to aromatherapy principles, a whiff of a citrus fruit or fresh mint can help you feel more alert, so make sure to inhale the next time you peel an orange, and try adding some fresh mint to your salad or a pitcher of water.[10]

- **Eat a piece of fruit**. The natural fruit sugars in fruits like bananas and apples can help lift energy levels.

- **Grab a handful of walnuts.** They won't give you a jolt of energy, but walnuts contain biotin, which helps you metabolize energy from the food you eat.

For some people, it's not so much the caffeine from coffee that they rely on, but the ritual of drinking a comforting warm beverage or a yummy iced drink. And some women find they need to drink something warm in the morning to have a "productive" trip to the bathroom. Here are some ideas for weaning yourself off caffeine and expanding your beverage horizons.

- **Go decaf.** Head to your favorite coffee place—the one with baristas you trust—and get your favorite drink made decaf. Explain to them that it's *really* important that it's decaf—not just for you, but for future generations of coffee addicts. Decaf green or black teas are also options. Both still have the antioxidants of the regular stuff, just without the kick.

- **Go half-caf–half-decaf.** If you can't go without (and there were some days I just couldn't), go with less. It works, and you'll be cutting back significantly on your caffeine intake. Then, try to wean yourself completely by adding less and less of the full-strength stuff to your mug.

- **Pick up a new habit.** Teecino is a caffeine-free, herbal "coffee." It's made from roasted and ground herbs, grains, fruits, and nuts. You brew it just like regular coffee, so you can still wake up to a nice aroma in the morning. As a bonus, it's rich in potassium.

- **Go red.** Herbal tea is always an option, but make sure the label says it's caffeine-free, and steer clear of any that contain herbal supplements, like St. John's wort. A great herbal tea to try is rooibos (also known as red tea), which comes from a type of bush that grows in South Africa and is packed with flavonoids. There's also a product out called Red Espresso, which you can make shots of—just like the real deal. I like it iced.

- **Try a tisane.** You've probably had a tisane at some point without even knowing it. A tisane is a tea-like beverage that doesn't contain any tea leaves from the *camellia sinensis* plant; instead, it's brewed with fruit (fresh or dried), herbs, flowers, or roots. You can make a tisane of ginger and lemon that's a really nice way to start your day. It's great for soothing morning sickness, it helps with digestion, and it also has a nice warming effect. I used it to kick my coffee habit during a trip to the Himalayas. Here's the recipe:

Ginger, Lemon, and Honey Tisane

Adapted from a recipe I discovered at Ananda,
a destination spa located in the Himalayas of India

Makes 1 pot

20 ounces water

1½ tablespoons chopped fresh ginger

1 tablespoon fresh lemon juice

2 tablespoons honey

1. Heat the water in a kettle until piping hot. Meanwhile, place the ginger, lemon juice, and honey in a heatproof teapot.
2. Pour the hot water over the other ingredients. Let steep for 3 minutes and serve.

Energy Drink Alert

If you're a fan of products with açai—that antioxidant-packed little rainforest berry from Brazil—take a good look at the product label and make sure it doesn't contain guarana extract or guarana berries. Açai drinks often include a hit of guarana (in Brazil, the two berries are traditionally used together) because guarana is used as an energy booster; that makes sense, because it contains quite a bit of caffeine. Case in point: A friend of mine once complained to me that she couldn't fall asleep at night. I asked her how much coffee or tea she was drinking, and she said she was drinking nothing but watered-down açai juice—all day long.

While it's not as caffeine-packed as coffee, the guarana in many açai products does have enough kick to be used as a stimulant. An 11.5-ounce bottle of açai juice with guarana has 55 mg caffeine, compared to 95 mg in a cup of coffee. Açai berries and their juice are a great way to get an antioxidant boost—just make sure what you're drinking or eating is guarana-free. I recommend skipping açai smoothies made at chain smoothie places because they use premixed powders and juice blends, and the server may not know exactly what's in them.

In fact, make sure to skip any of the energy-boost powders you can add to your smoothie—they're likely to contain some kind of stimulant. Yerba mate is another caffeine-packed herb that's being used in all sorts of drinks. Look out for the word "energy" on bottled juices, teas, and smoothies—chances are the product contains green tea extract, yerba mate, ginseng, or guarana, all of which are stimulants.

Belly Tip

Get juicy. If you're trying to cut back on artificial sweeteners and processed sugars—definitely a good idea—you might be struggling to find a more natural way to sweeten drinks. Apple juice (go for organic) can be added to herbal tea and sparkling water. It blends right in with your beverage; you don't even need to mix it.

Three Cheers for Chocolate

But hey, look on the bright side: you can still enjoy chocolate! Yes, the food of the gods does contain a little caffeine, but much less than caffeinated beverages (see the chart starting on the next page), and it can be a great mood lifter. In fact, a study done a few years ago at the University of Helsinki found that babies of moms who ate chocolate daily were more active and smiled and laughed more often. Even moms who considered themselves under stress had babies who were more chilled out than the infants of stressed moms who didn't eat chocolate.[11]

There's even more good news for chocolate during pregnancy. A study done by researchers at Yale and the University of California found that women who ate chocolate while pregnant had a reduced risk of preeclampsia. The researchers didn't just take the participants' word for how much chocolate (in the form of dark or milk chocolate, cocoa, chocolate milk, chocolate cake, cookies, or ice cream) they ate; they also tested the levels of theobromine—a plant chemical in chocolate that's similar to caffeine and crosses the placenta—in their umbilical cord blood. Theobromine doesn't have as much of a stimulating effect on the nervous system as caffeine, and it actually lowers blood pressure. It has been used to treat hypertension, angina, and atherosclerosis. The results: Women who ate the most chocolate (five servings or more per week) and whose babies had the highest concentration of theobromine in their cord blood were 69 percent less likely to develop preeclampsia. The beneficial effect of chocolate seemed to be most important during the last three months of pregnancy.[12]

This news ranks right up there with the discovery that your high school rival is living in a trailer park. Before you go to Costco and start buying Hershey's bars in bulk, keep in mind that a 1.3-ounce bar of chocolate contains about 200 calories. Dark chocolate has a little less sugar than milk chocolate and contains more theobromine, so it's a smarter choice. Oh, and if you're a white chocolate fan: Sorry, it doesn't contain any of the plant chemicals that make chocolate good for you.[13]

One final note: If you've been diagnosed with gestational diabetes, talk to your doctor before adding any sweets to your diet.

Caffeine Content of Foods and Beverages[14]

8-ounce cup of coffee	95 to 200 mg
14 dark chocolate-covered coffee beans	138 mg
16-ounce chai latte	100 mg

1 can Red Bull	80 mg
12-ounce can Jolt Cola	71.5 mg
1-ounce espresso shot	64 mg
1 cup coffee ice cream	58 mg
8-ounce cup of black tea	47 mg
1 serving instant cappuccino	39 mg
12-ounce can of cola	29 mg
8-ounce cup of green tea	25 mg
8-ounce cup of white tea	20 mg
1 1.69-ounce bag of milk chocolate M&Ms	7 mg
6-ounce cup of instant cocoa	4 mg
8-ounce low-fat chocolate milk	2 mg

Source: USDA National Nutrient Database for Standard Reference, The Tea Council, wetplanet.com, and CSPI (Center for Science in the Public Interest)

Cheese and Milk

The advice on cheese used to be that if it wasn't hard, you shouldn't touch it (but isn't that what got you into your current state?). Then in 2003, the Food and Drug Administration (FDA) made a slight change to their advice. Instead of recommending that all soft cheeses should be avoided, now they say you just can't eat unpasteurized—or raw—soft cheeses.[15] The issue with raw-milk cheese (and raw milk itself) is that it could contain *Listeria monocytogenes* (there's a ton more on this fun subject on page 124), a bacteria that is extremely dangerous for pregnant women because it can lead to miscarriage.

I don't know about you, but I never gave cheese that much thought. Do the packages say "pasteurized"? I had no idea. To be safe, if the label doesn't specifically say that it's pasteurized, don't put it in your basket.

To make matters even more confusing, both soft and hard cheeses can be made from raw (unpasteurized) milk. You're more likely to find these types of cheeses at gourmet stores than at run-of-the-mill grocery stores. Since so many foodies are now on the hunt for raw-milk cheeses, stores are carrying even more options than ever. I practically had to bring a decoder ring with me when shopping at my upscale neighborhood market during my pregnancy.

So what about a soufflé or a casserole that's made with unpasteurized cheese? Would that be okay? I posed this question to the Food and Drug Administration and the Partnership for Food Safety Education. They responded that it would be safe for a pregnant woman to eat if heated to 165°F or above. However, to avoid any potential cross-contamination (such as chopping lettuce on the same board where your hubby crumbled the blue cheese), it's wiser still to keep those rogue cheeses out of your fridge altogether.

Belly Tip

Sneaky cheese. If you're at a restaurant where you suspect the cheese might be unpasteurized, ask your server to talk to the chef and find out for sure. Another thing to keep in mind is that lots of salads—such as Cobb and spinach salads—often include blue cheese or gorgonzola. It's not always listed on the menu description; unfortunately, I spaced out about this several times during my first few weeks of pregnancy.

Naughty*	Nice
Blue	American
Brie	Cheddar
Camembert	Jarlsberg
Feta	Swiss
Fresh mozzarella	Cheese slices

* Remember, if it's made with pasteurized milk—and I've found a lot of feta, gorgonzola, and fresh mozzarella that are—it's safe!

Gorgonzola	Cheese spreads (However, these are high in fat, so make sure to read the label.)
Limburger	Semi-soft cheeses: cream cheese, cottage cheese, and ricotta
Fresh Mexican–style cheeses (queso blanco, queso fresco)	Shredded, packaged cheese blends (Mexican-blend shredded cheeses in ziplock bags are fine, too.)

Juice

What's wrong with a little roadside apple cider, you ask? While it's certainly tasty, it might not be pasteurized. The pasteurization process briefly heats juices to a high temperature, which kills off any potential bacteria or parasites that could be lurking. Pretty much all the juices you'll find in your grocery store are pasteurized. You'll see the untreated stuff at farm stands and health-food stores.[16] This note is of special concern when you're traveling internationally: Don't expect *mango liquado* at a roadside stand in Tegucigalpa, Guatemala, to be made from pasteurized juice.

This doesn't mean that if a juice is cloudy, you should always skip it. A juice can be pasteurized *and* unfiltered, which just means it has sediment in it. The sediment gives it a cloudy appearance. In fact, unfiltered apple juice is actually a healthier choice.

Belly Tip

Cut the kombucha. Kombucha is a fermented tea that's become very popular recently. It's got a vinegar or pickle-juice flavor, and it's teeming with bacteria. This is good when you're not pregnant and need some help reestablishing levels of probiotics. But kombucha isn't pasteurized, so it can harbor potentially harmful bacteria.[17] Definitely don't try to make your own home brew. Skip the kombucha for now, and get your good bugs with the probiotic sources I mention on page 94.

Wieners, Lox, and More

One of the things that *really* disappointed me was learning that lox and other smoked and refrigerated seafood was on the don't-go-there-during-pregnancy list. Ladies who like their ballpark franks will be bummed to know that unless they're served super-steaming hot, hot dogs are to be shunned as well. And you *foie gras* fans are out of luck, too, because refrigerated meat pâtés and spreads are contraband. But if you want, you *can* eat all the Spam or other canned meat you want.

Huh? Sounds odd, right? Well, the stuff in cans is shelf-stable, which means that nothing can grow in it. Refrigerated products are more susceptible to the growth of bacteria unless they are strictly kept below 40°F.[18] But unless you find yourself stranded in a cabin in the woods, I'd avoid the shelf-stable versions of pâté and meat spreads because they're ridiculously high in sodium and nitrates.

One of the most confusing, annoying, and tough to remember things that you shouldn't have during pregnancy is deli meat. Nope—not even the organic, nitrate-free variety. Why the hell not? Well, it's all about keeping the meat at the right temperature. The issue with deli meats, like turkey, ham, bologna, and chicken breast is that, just like raw cheese, they are prone to *listeria*. *Listeria* is particularly tricky because it can grow at low temperatures, so even if you've been keeping your cold cuts in the fridge, they can still be susceptible.

The reason why *listeria* and other foodborne illnesses are such a concern for you right now is that your immune system takes a hit while you're pregnant. Bacteria that your body may have been able to fend off before may now find you to be a much more hospitable host. That little one you're carrying doesn't have a developed immune system yet, so she can't fight anything off. And unfortunately, foodborne bacteria can cross the placenta and cause harm to your baby.[19]

Think about it: Do you really think that sub shop or corner deli is keeping its smoked turkey below 33°F? Probably not. Now, if you wanted, you could heat up that turkey sandwich till it's a piping 165°F, making it safe to eat. But I don't trust that the angsty teen behind the counter is going to use a meat thermometer on my hoagie, and honestly, I prefer my turkey sandwich cold.

Raw and Uncooked Foods

Tuna carpaccio, cookie dough, bean sprouts, and Caesar salad (if it's made with raw egg) are all delicious, but all have a risk of carrying bacteria.[20] The good news is that there's not a huge list of foods made with raw ingredients (but raw, unwashed fruits and vegetables also carry some risk). In fact, in France, where many women still drink wine fairly regularly during pregnancy, doctors advise their patients to avoid salad. Ah, cultural differences. For more on how to keep all that fresh stuff safe, turn to page 126 in "Chapter 14: Germ Patrol."

Seafood

There are four types of fish that you should completely kick to the curb before, during, and after pregnancy (if you breast-feed): swordfish, tilefish, king mackerel, and shark. Swordfish is the most common of these, but I've been seeing tilefish on menus more frequently lately.[21]

Fresh tuna has not been part of the no-no list, but the *New York Times* sounded alarm bells concerning methyl mercury levels in tuna sushi in a 2008 article. The *Times* tested samples of high-end restaurant and take-out tuna from many New York City restaurants. Of the forty-four samples, eight had mercury levels high enough to be pulled off the shelves by the EPA. More than half of the samples were high enough in mercury that consuming only six pieces per week would be more than what is safe for the average person (who the EPA says weighs 154 pounds; people who weigh less should consume even less mercury). Some of the tuna samples were from bluefin tuna, which has higher mercury levels than other types of tuna.[22] Bottom line: Avoid sushi, especially tuna, and since you can't cook away methyl mercury, it's smart to avoid tuna steaks as well.

What about the canned stuff? Smaller fish are generally used for canned tuna (it's all going to get chopped up anyway), and smaller fish have smaller amounts of mercury. Albacore (often referred to as white) tuna is higher in mercury than chunk light tuna, so if you're craving a tuna-fish sandwich, make it at home with chunk light tuna. The EPA says that you can eat as much as 6 ounces (one can) of albacore tuna per week when you're pregnant,[23] but I say, why not skip the risk and stick with chunk light? Of course, if you have a craving for a tuna-fish sandwich at a restaurant and aren't sure which kind it uses, go for it.

It's a bummer if you love oysters, but all raw seafood should be avoided when you're expecting. A nasty bacteria called *vibrio* (see page 126) can contaminate shellfish, especially oysters. *Vibrio* is more common during the warm summer months, which is why it's recommended to eat raw oysters only in months ending in "ber," like September and October. Proper cooking kills the bacteria, but steaming (like at an oyster roast) might not be enough to do the trick.[24]

If you happen to live near a lake, river, or the ocean and actually catch some of your own fish (or have nice neighbors who do), make sure to follow your local advisories. Even with all these concerns, seafood is an important food for pregnant women. For more on choosing fish that's safe, turn to page 69 for the "Go Fish" chapter.

Artificial Sweeteners

This is a hot-button topic for many people. It seems like some folks have as much allegiance to their little blue or yellow packets of sweetener as they do to their political parties. Using that analogy, here's the official party line:

According to the Food and Drug Administration, acesulfame potassium (Sunett), sucralose (Splenda), and aspartame (Equal, NutraSweet) are safe to use during pregnancy. The caveat with the last one is that if you have phenylketonuria, or if you have high levels of phenylalanine in your blood, you should steer clear, because the sweetener won't metabolize properly (turn to page 119 for more on phenylketonuria).[25]

On the absolute no-no list is saccharin (Sweet'N Low). And even though it was recently declared safe by the FDA, I'd be cautious about using stevia.[26, 27] Stevia is a natural sweetener that comes from the leaves of the *Stevia rebaudiana* plant. It's 250 times sweeter than table sugar. Recently, it's become very popular and is being used to sweeten beverages. Some people love the taste of it and have switched over to using stevia because it's more natural than most calorie-free sweeteners. But it hasn't been tested on pregnant women, so either avoid it or limit your consumption of products sweetened with stevia (or Truvia, Sweet Simplicity, or PureVia). If you have switched over to stevia, you may want to go back to regular old sugar, or give honey a try. It has just as many calories, but it's all-natural and not processed.

Ultimately, whether you choose to use one of the approved artificial sweeteners or not is a very individual choice. Personally, I don't touch the stuff. Several studies have shown that artificial sweeteners do not help you lose weight. I'd rather burn off 21 calories in a teaspoon of honey, or 16 calories in a teaspoon of sugar, than add more chemicals to my diet.

The one exception? Chewing gum. It just doesn't make sense to keep something packed with sugar in your mouth for that long.

Unripe Papaya

Papaya, when it's ripe and a rich orange color, is a healthy, folate-rich fruit. When unripe (aka green), however, it contains a latex substance that can trigger uterine contractions. The latex found in unripe papaya acts like oxytocin and prostaglandin, which are both hormones involved in labor.[28]

Black Licorice

Strange as it sounds, real black licorice candy (made with licorice root extract), or licorice root used as a supplement, may increase the risk of preterm labor. Glycyrrhizin—the substance that gives licorice its sweet taste—also seems to cause preterm labor. A study done in Finland in 2002 found that women who ate high amounts of black licorice (more than a pound a week) were more than two times as likely to go into preterm labor (earlier than thirty-seven weeks).[29] I'm a huge black licorice fan (candy, tea, anything) and find it helps to soothe an upset stomach. But to be on the safe side, skip it when you're preggers. Take heart, Twizzlers fans—the cherry, strawberry, and chocolate flavored varieties don't contain any licorice extract at all.[30]

Herbal Remedies

They might seem like the most natural thing to turn to for your pregnancy-induced symptoms, but many herbal supplements are off limits during pregnancy because their safety hasn't been tested on pregnant women. Herbal supplements are now used in many food products and over-the-counter remedies, however, so you have to really be on the lookout.

Herbs that should be avoided are:[31]
Saw palmetto
Goldenseal
Ephedra
Comfrey
Yohimbe
Pay d'arco
Passion flower
Black cohosh
Blue cohosh
Roman chamomile
Pennyroyal
Willow bark (it contains the same chemical component as aspirin)

Spa Safety

I highly recommend indulging in spa treatments during your pregnancy, but you have to be careful about using essential oils. Essential oils are the concentrated aromatic part of plants. They're generally mixed with other oils like sesame, avocado, and grapeseed oil (and they should never be applied to the skin undiluted). Once mixed, they're used in "aromatherapy" treatments, including massage, facials, manicures, and pedicures, to help relieve tension or perk you up.[32]

Make sure you see a licensed massage therapist or aesthetician (I ran into a few who didn't know diddly about what to avoid) who is familiar with which essential oils are safe to use during pregnancy. Some are highly potent and can cause uterine contractions. Oils to avoid during pregnancy—especially during the first and second trimester—are clary sage, geranium, cypress, juniper, and rosemary. In fact, some women use clary sage during labor to help bring on contractions.[33]

According to Dawn Bierschwal, owner of the Becoming Mom Spa in Mason, Ohio, it's a better idea to buy essential oils specifically formulated for pregnancy rather than making your own. She likes the ones from Mama Mio (www.mamamio.com) and Naturopathica (www.naturopathica.com). If you're confused about which oils are safe, call the customer-care line and speak to an expert. Or you can play it completely safe and ask for a massage without any essential oils (that's what I do at my local nail place).

According to Bierschwal, the following oils are safe to use during pregnancy, but should still be used in small amounts:[34]

Oil	Benefit
Lavender	Antiseptic, relaxing
Lemongrass	Aids circulation
Mandarin	Diuretic; used in foot treatments to help with puffiness
Neroli	Tension relief
Tea tree oil	Antiseptic
Ylang ylang	Aphrodesiac, so good for preconception; relaxation

About Those Plastic Bottles...

No doubt you've added drinking from reusable plastic bottles to your list of things to freak out about. Here's the deal. Environmental groups have been concerned over the safety of bisphenol A (BPA), a chemical used in polycarbonate plastics, for some time. BPA makes plastic durable and shatter-resistant and is used in products like baby bottles, reusable sports bottles, and the linings of food, drink, and baby formula cans. In spring 2008, the Department of Health and Human Services' National Toxicology Program found that exposure to BPA could have adverse neural and behavioral effects on fetuses, babies, and children. Canada has banned BPA outright.[35]

What can you do? The good news is that there are now plenty of options that are chemical-free for both you and your baby. Ditch transparent bottles with a PC (for polycarbonate) stamp on the bottom of the bottle, and go for ones made by Camel-Bak or old-school (not clear) polyethylene ones by Nalgene. You may choose to switch to an aluminum water bottle, like ones made by Sigg or Klean Kanteen. You should also avoid eating canned foods often and drinking sodas, as the linings of cans contain BPA.

Once your baby arrives, use BPA-free bottles, such as those made by Born Free, zoë b, Adiri, and Green to Grow. Sippy cups and baby bowls come BPA-free too. Yes, they're a bit more pricey, but it's definitely worth it. And now that large retailers like Wal-Mart and Toys "R" Us (Babies "R" Us, too) are banning BPA, it's only a matter of time before the chemical is phased out of products completely.[36]

Okay, there you go—that's the worst of it. If you're like me, you'll spend a lot of time looking at menus for a while, mentally crossing off all the things you can't have, but it gets easier and more automatic to avoid those questionable foods over time. And all these small changes to stay safe now will add up to a whole lot of confidence that your baby will be healthy and happy.

Chapter Six

The Big O
(Organic, That Is)

As a soon-to-be momma, you want to treat your body as well as you possibly can. One way to help ensure that is by eating organic. After all, you're sharing everything you eat and drink with your little one.

While not many studies have been done on the effect of pesticides on pregnant women (you can imagine why), some research does point an ugly finger at the detrimental results of common pesticide use. An Indiana University School of Medicine Study in May 2007 found that premature births increased during the months that pesticides and nitrate (used to fertilize crops and lawns) residues in surface water (including drinking water) are highest—April to July—and the rates were lowest in months when the residues were least detectable (August to September).[1]

The lead researcher—a neonatologist— explained that nitrates can wreak havoc on the endocrine system of a developing fetus and may cause early labor. Scary stuff, right? What does this mean for you? Other than inducing labor or scheduling a C-section, there's not much you can do about when your baby will be born.

But you can help reduce your exposure by avoiding the biggest sources of pesticides and other chemicals in your food and in your home. It's wonderful to be vigilant about your health, but at the same time, you're also trying to save your pennies for Junior. Make a compromise, and buy organic for those items that matter the most. Of course, if you have the cash and the inclination, feel free to go all organic.

Organic dairy is free from pesticides and the hormones and antibiotics that most conventional dairy cows are treated with. And now there's even more reason to buy organic milk and yogurt. A study at Newcastle University in the United Kingdom found that milk from organically raised cows was higher in fatty acids (the good-for-you kind), antioxidants, and vitamins than milk from conventionally raised cows.[2] Organic milk is rich in conjugated linoleic acid (CLA), a type of omega-3 fatty acid that has been linked to inhibiting cancer, lowering bad cholesterol, improving immune function, enhancing bone building, and even improving the use of glucose in diabetics (some of these benefits have only been shown in the lab). Organic cows produced 60 percent more good fat in the summer months, when grass and clover supplies were at their peak.[3] It just goes to show that what animals eat affects their milk, just like what you eat affects your milk (for more on the link between diet and the quality of your breast milk, turn to page 256). Kind of a no-brainer, huh? Because CLA is a component of milk fat, you won't find it in skim milk; that's another reason why I generally call for organic 1% milk in my recipes.

Organically raised meat and poultry are better for you for the same reasons as organic dairy. According to the USDA organic regulations, meat that is labeled "organic" must come from animals that haven't been treated with hormones (to make them bigger) or with antibiotics (to try to keep them disease free).[4] Of course that's not to say that I never ate nonorganic meat or dairy when I was pregnant (I am a food editor, after all), but I tried to choose it at home or whenever the choice was available.

Veg Out

One of the best things you can do for yourself when you're pregnant or trying to get preggers is eat tons of fruits and vegetables. The U.S. government recommends 2 cups of fruit and 2½ cups of vegetables a day, which comes out to a total of 9 servings in a 2,000-calorie diet. Most of us can't live up to that. And it's not the easiest thing in the world to do—you actually have to plan for it. But more on that later.

You want to load up on fresh produce, but you're also concerned about pesticides, right? Well, chemical residue is a bigger issue for some fruits and vegetables than others. In general, the thicker the skin on the produce, the harder it is for pesticides to affect the part you eat.

Use the list below, developed by the Environmental Working Group (EWG) (or download your very own from EWG's site, foodnews.org), to know when you should pony up the extra money for organics or choose conventional. They say that by avoiding the so-called "dirty dozen" and opting for the least-sprayed produce, you can cut your exposure to pesticides by 90 percent. It's a great thing to get acquainted with now, because you'll want to follow the same rules when Baby starts eating solids.[5]

Go Organic

- **Peaches**.

- **Apples**. These fruits are really something you should snack on daily, with the skin. Not only does that crunchy outside have a lot of fiber, it's also where much of the nutrients are—namely, quercitin. This tough-to-pronounce phytochemical (plant-based chemical) is in the class of flavonoids and has anti-inflammatory and antioxidant benefits. A recent study found that eating apples during pregnancy reduced the risk of having a child with asthma or childhood wheezing.

- **Sweet bell peppers**.
- **Celery**.
- **Nectarines**.
- **Strawberries**.
- **Cherries**.

- **Lettuce**.
- **Grapes** (imported).
- **Pears**.
- **Spinach**.
- **Potatoes**.

Conventional Is Okay

- **Onions**.
- **Avocado**.
- **Sweet corn** (frozen).
- **Pineapples**.
- **Mango**.
- **Sweet peas** (frozen).
- **Asparagus**.
- **Kiwi**.
- **Bananas**.
- **Cabbage**.
- **Broccoli**.
- **Eggplant**.
- **Papaya**.
- **Grapefruit**.
- **Watermelon**.
- **Honeydew melon**.
- **Lemon**.

Belly Tip

Kick 'em off. I always thought that people who made you take your shoes off before entering their home were over-the-top anal. I mean, what's a little dirt, right? Here's the deal: We track in *everything* on our shoes, from the herbicide that your neighbor uses on her lawn to the gasoline you put in your Prius. Not such a huge deal, but then those chemicals become airborne in household dust, making them just the right size to inhale. So drop your shoes just outside your front or back door. You'll be keeping your floors—and your lungs—much cleaner.

What About Local?

There's been a ton of recent hype about local food being even better for you than organic. Well, it totally depends. If you're buying produce on the least-sprayed list, it's probably better to go for something that was locally grown, because it didn't have to travel as far, lose as many nutrients along the way, or waste all that greenhouse gas-producing gasoline. Local produce that you'd buy at your farmers market or grocery store (look for a sign saying that it's locally grown) doesn't sit out nearly as long as food that's been trucked cross-country. The longer fruits and vegetables sit around before you eat them, the more nutrients they lose due to heat and light damage.

Just remember that local produce may still be sprayed with pesticides. The cool thing about shopping for local produce—especially at your farmers market or co-op—is that you can talk to the farmer directly about how the food is grown. Growers also give you great tips on what's in season, and how to use and store it.

Chapter Seven

Go Fish

If you're utterly confused about whether you should be eating seafood at all during your pregnancy, join the crowd. When the Food and Drug Administration and Environmental Protection Agency released their original joint advisory on seafood and pregnancy in 2004, it was a great public service and helped steer women away from the major food sources of harmful methyl mercury: shark, swordfish, tilefish, and king mackerel.[1] Unfortunately, the media hysteria that followed caused many women to misinterpret the advice and stop eating seafood altogether. Many of my pregnant (and about-to-be-pregnant) friends told me they had sworn off seafood because it was just too hard to keep track of what was on the okay list and what wasn't. I'm hoping this chapter will help clear up the confusion and help you make an easy choice the next time you're at a restaurant or at the seafood counter in the grocery store.

My mother always told me that fish was "brain food," and to my preteen mind, that sounded pretty gross. But just as she was about so many other things, Mom was actually right. The fatty acids in seafood, docosahexanoic acid (DHA) and eicosapentaenoic acid (EPA) (both forms of omega-3), have been shown to play a key role in the development of a baby's brain. The Food and Drug Administration and Environmental Protection Agency recommend that pregnant women eat up to 12 ounces of low-mercury fish and shellfish a week. So fish is good for pregnant women, right?

Yes, and no.

According to Dr. Steve Otwell, a professor at the School of Food Science and Nutrition at the University of Florida, "Even the small risk that can come from a lifetime of exposure to mercury is outweighed by the immediate and essential benefits."[2] Yes, certain fish should be avoided, but the experts all agree that the benefits of seafood to your baby greatly outweigh the risk. The National Healthy Mothers, Healthy Babies Coalition, a group made up of professors of obstetrics and PhDs in nutrition, announced in October 2007 that women who want to become pregnant, pregnant women, and women who are breast-feeding should eat *no less than* 12 ounces of seafood a week.[3] So that flatly goes up against the FDA warnings to eat *no more than* 12 ounces. They also emphasized that selenium—a mineral naturally occurring in ocean fish—appears to protect against toxicity from trace amounts of mercury.

The science continues to build a case for ladies with a bun to sidle up to the seafood counter. A 2007 paper published in the *Lancet* by Dr. Joseph R. Hibbeln found that women with a low seafood intake (less than 12 ounces a week) had children who scored lower on tests for fine motor, communication, and social development skills from ages six months to eight years. He also found that when women ate more than the government-recommended 12 ounces a week, their children's neurodevelopment and verbal IQ scores benefited.[4] The study was performed in the United Kingdom, which has higher methyl mercury-exposure levels than the United States does. So once again the researchers concluded that the benefits of that filet o' fish or salmon salad are greater than skipping them.

What's so fantastic about fish? DHA is the mack daddy for your baby's brain and eye development. DHA is an omega-3 polyunsaturated fat that's an essential fatty acid, which means our bodies don't make it and we need to get it from the food we eat. It's found mainly in fatty cold-water fish, like salmon, herring, tuna, trout, mackerel (typically Atlantic mackerel, not king mackerel, which is on the don't-eat list), and oysters. It's also found in organ meats (such as liver) and breast milk. DHA is also now being added to everything from orange juice, yogurt, and soy milk (good), to chocolates (a little too fishy tasting).

DHA plays a key role in the development of a growing fetus' brain and neurological system. Your baby is dependent on you to supply her with enough DHA. That means that if you don't get an adequate amount for both of you, your stores can become depleted, especially while you're breast-feeding. Unfortunately, most pregnant and breast-feeding women only get about 50 mg a day of DHA.[5] Make sure to get 200 mg a day while you're pregnant and also throughout breast-feeding.

Here are some of the top seafood sources of omega-3 (per 3-ounce serving):[6]

Anchovies★	2,055 mg
Atlantic salmon, farmed	1,800 mg
Salmon, wild coho	900 mg
Sardines	982 mg
Chunk light tuna	200 mg
Catfish, farmed	200 mg
Atlantic cod	100 mg
Pollock	500 mg
Scallops	300 mg
Crab	400 mg
Shrimp	300 mg
Tilapia★★	135 mg
Kona kampachi (also called hamachi):	1740 mg

Sources: International Food Information Council,
educational booklet on Fish and Your Health; nal.usda.gov

★   Per 3.5 ounce serving—Note: this is a heck of a lot of anchovies! You can eat much less and still get a benefit. Try them on pizza.
★★ Per 3.5 ounce serving

Another benefit of omega-3 in both the DHA and EPA forms is that it helps protect against mood disorders, such as depression and bipolar disorder.[7] Low levels of DHA in breast milk and low seafood consumption levels have been linked to postpartum depression, which affects 10 to 15 percent of mothers.[8] Taking a combination of DHA and EPA has been shown in some studies to significantly improve the symptoms of postpartum depression.[9]

To top it all off, seafood is also great for your heart. In 2006, the American Heart Association released a statement encouraging Americans to eat two servings a week of fish—preferably the fatty kind, like salmon and herring.[10]

Need more reasons to eat fish? A recent study found that the children of mothers who ate fish during pregnancy had a lower risk of eczema.[11] A Harvard study by Emily Oken found that moms who ate the most fish had kids who performed better on cognitive tests at age three, while moms with higher mercury levels had kids with poorer test scores.[12] Basically, this means you need to maximize your fish intake while minimizing your mercury exposure. So which fish are the better catch? Seafood with low or no detectable levels of mercury include the following:[13]

- **Catfish.** Although, unless you were raised on it, you're probably not going to be eating a heck of a lot of this one.

- **Pollock.** It's the white fish used to make "imitation crab" and fish fillets at fast-food joints.

- **Shrimp.** Probably because it's so easy to prepare, shrimp has now surpassed tuna as the most popular seafood in America. Go for shrimp bearing a "Wild American" seal—recently, shrimp imported from China and Vietnam were found to be contaminated with antibiotics. At restaurants, ask your server where the shrimp were caught; you can also check out a list of restaurants that serve Wild American shrimp at www.wildamericanshrimp.com.

- **Salmon.** Next to anchovies, salmon is the richest source of omega-3. Plus, it's easy to make and fairly versatile. The only downside is that it has become overfished. Curious why farmed salmon is richer in omega-3 than wild? It's because it has more fat overall. Farmed fish move around less than their leaner, wild counterparts.

- **Tilapia.** A mild, sweet-fleshed fish, tilapia is great in fish tacos or pan-seared and served with vegetables.

- **Kona kampachi.** Also known as hamachi or Hawaiian yellowtail, this farmed fish from Hawaii is sweet and meaty. It's been showing up on menus at a lot of top restaurants. It has undetectable levels of contaminants and is rich in omega-3.

If you're concerned about overfishing (and really, we all should be), download a Seafood Watch wallet card from the Monterey Bay Aquarium's website at http://www.mbayaq.org/cr/cr_seafoodwatch/download.asp. It'll tell you which fish to go for and which to avoid based on both human health and the health of the oceans.[14] There's a national version that anyone can use, and they also have regional guides that address specific overfishing concerns in your area.

Non-Fishy DHA

What if you're vegetarian, vegan, or just not into eating stuff from the sea? There are plenty of new fortified products on the market with added DHA. Of course, getting nutrients from natural food sources is always the best route, but here are some other ways to get what you need:

- **Omega-3 supplements.** These offer various amounts of DHA and EPA. One I like is Solgar Omega-3 "950." Each softgel contains 408 mg of DHA and 542 mg of EPA sourced from cold-water fish. As with most pills, it's smart to take omega-3s on a full stomach to avoid nausea. Some people find that they burp up the pills, which— as you can imagine—is rather unpleasant. Start out with a small bottle (they're pricey) and see how you do with them. Also, several prenatal vitamins are fortified with DHA these days. Prescription-only Prenate DHA and PrimaCare ONE both contain more than 200 mg of DHA per capsule. Over-the-counter brand One-a-Day Women's Prenatal contains 200 mg of DHA per pill.

- **Juices.** If you drink an 8-ounce glass of DHA-fortified orange juice, such as Tropicana Healthy Heart, you're getting 50 mg of a combination of DHA and EPA sourced from fish oil and fish gelatin. It sounds absolutely vile, but it tastes just like regular O.J.

- **Eggs.** DHA-fortified eggs—from companies like Gold Circle Farms—come from chickens that have been fed a special vegetarian DHA-rich diet, and that comes through in their eggs. Each egg boasts 150 mg of DHA, versus 18 mg in a regular egg.

- **Dairy products.** One 8-ounce glass of DHA-fortified milk from Horizon Organic has 32 mg of DHA from a vegetarian source (algae). Now, several yogurt companies are packing those little cups full of brain-boosting omega-3. Rachel's offers yogurt in unique flavors, such as Pink Grapefruit Lychee. The company's yogurts contain an algal form of DHA—32 mg of it per serving. Breyers also makes an omega-3 fortified yogurt called Fruit-on-the-Bottom Smart!, which is also enhanced with DHA from algae.

- **Specialty products.** DHA-fortified pregnancy foods like Bellybars, Bellybar chews, and Bellybar shakes boast 50 mg of DHA per serving (also sourced from algae). The citrus chews are my favorite, because you can keep them in your purse. They taste like Starburst candies! Oh! Mama bars have 150 mg of algae-sourced DHA.

- **Chocolate.** Various companies have tried putting DHA from both fish and algae into chocolate. Maybe it's because I'm a chocolate purist, but I can always taste that subtle hint o' mackerel in these products. Chocolate just shouldn't be messed with, in my book. Why not have a lovely salmon fillet followed by a single, amazing chocolate truffle for dessert? That's *my* choice.

Chapter Eight

How to Deal When You're Meat-Free, Dairy-Free, or Wheat-Free

If you're vegetarian or vegan, you're in good company these days. According to a survey by *Vegetarian Times* magazine, 7.3 million Americans—3.2 percent of U.S adults —are vegetarians. About a million of them follow a vegan diet.[1] It's probably not a big surprise to you that there are more meat-free women than men—59 percent of vegetarians are women.

Like Stella McCartney, you can have a perfectly healthy pregnancy and stick to your meat-free ways. It just takes a bit more effort. But if you've been following a vegetarian lifestyle for a while, you're probably used to going the extra mile. Your biggest concern will be getting enough iron, protein, calcium, and vitamin B_{12} in your diet. But a prenatal vitamin can help cover your bases.

Get Pumped

As I mentioned in "Chapter 2: Baby Bonuses and Momma Must-Haves," vitamin C helps you absorb iron. So team up iron-rich vegetarian foods with ones rich in C. Remember, the goal is to get 27 to 30 mg of iron each day.

Vegetarian sources of iron:[2]

1 cup fortified cereal (Total Raisin Bran)	18 mg
1 cup cooked spinach	6.43 mg
1 cup instant fortified oatmeal	3.96 mg

1 cup cooked Swiss chard	3.95 mg
1 cup dried apricots	3.46 mg
½ cup tofu	3.35 mg
1 cup canned kidney beans	3.25 mg
1 cup dried figs	3 mg
½ cup raisins	1.5 mg
1 small baked potato with skin	1.49 mg
1 cup cooked kale	1.17 mg
1 cup cooked broccoli	1.12 mg

Source: nal.usda.gov

I have to just throw this out there—many vegetarians experience strong cravings for meat once they're pregnant. When I worked in a health-food store back in high school, I remember the manager telling me that she had been completely veg for years, but when she was pregnant, her red-meat cravings became so strong that she had to give in. If you find yourself jonesing for a little roast beef or a burger, your body most likely needs it. Think of it as a temporary walk on the dark side for a very good cause.

If your doctor finds that you have low iron levels, she may advise you to take supplements. Just remember to keep up your fiber intake so you don't get constipated, and drink plenty of water. Since iron supplements can also give you heartburn, make sure to take them with meals and never right before bed.

Belly Tip

Iron-clad rules. Coffee (not that you're drinking much these days), tea, egg yolks, milk, fiber, and soy protein can block iron absorption, so try to avoid them when you're eating iron-rich foods. Of course, if you're eating tofu, there's not much you can do about that.

No Moo

I'll skip the political debate over dairy and just say this: Dairy products are a great source of calcium and protein, but if you don't like them or can't tolerate them (many women can't as they get older), it's perfectly fine to do without. That said, you still need 1,000 mg of calcium each day. So how are you going to do that? Fill up on dairy-free foods that are rich in calcium and take a 500 mg calcium supplement each day.

Non-dairy, calcium-rich foods:[3]

1 cup fortified cereal (Total Raisin Bran)	1,000 mg
1 cup cooked spinach	245 mg
1 cup cooked Swiss chard	102 mg
1 cup cooked kale	94 mg
1 cup cooked broccoli	61 mg
1 cup black beans	46 mg
1 cup dried figs	241 mg
2 tablespoons tahini (sesame seed paste)	128 mg
1 ounce almonds	82 mg
2 tablespoons almond butter	86 mg
Tofu (look for calcium sulfate in the ingredient list)	861 mg
Calcium-fortified soy milk	300 mg
Calcium-fortified orange juice	350 mg

Source: nal.usda.gov

If you're dairy-free because you're lactose-intolerant, you might want to give cultured dairy products and yogurt a try. Because they have lower amounts of lactose (the sugar that causes all those gastric woes), they're often easier to digest than milk.

A lot of grown women shudder at the thought of drinking a glass of milk, but I actually suddenly found that a cold glass of milk sounded pretty damn good when I was pregnant. Unlike lots of other authors out there, I'm not going to tell you to choke it down. I will say that you can disguise milk (both cow and soy) in many more palatable ways. Here are a few ideas:

- Hot chocolate.

- Decaf latte.

- Chocolate milk.

- Chocolate and rice pudding.

- Smoothies (like the Nana-Berry Smoothie on page 249).

- Foods boosted with dried milk powder, like pancakes, soups, and baked goods.

Protein Punch

Those 60 grams of protein that you need each day can seem more elusive if you're vegetarian, especially if you're vegan. Try to fit a few of these foods into your diet each day.

Vegetarian sources of protein:

1 cup low-fat cottage cheese	28 grams
5.3-ounce cup Greek-style yogurt	15 grams
(Greek yogurt is strained, making it thicker, richer in protein, and lower in lactose)	
8-ounce cup plain yogurt	12 grams
Low-fat mozzarella string cheese	8 grams
Hardboiled egg	6 grams

Source: nal.usda.gov, HorizonOrganic.com, and OikosOrganic.com

Vegan sources of protein:[4]

1 cup edamame	29 grams
½ cup tofu	20 grams
1 veggie burger	18 grams
¼ cup soynuts	17 grams
½ cup tempeh	15 grams
1 cup black beans	15 grams
1 cup cooked quinoa	8 grams
2 tablespoons peanut butter	8 grams
1 ounce almonds	6 grams
2 tablespoons almond butter	5 grams

Source: nal.usda.gov, HorizonOrganic.com, and OikosOrganic.com

B Smart

Back in "Chapter 2: Baby Bonuses and Momma Must-Haves," I talked about the importance of vitamin B_{12} for baby's neurologic development. This is one nutrient that's definitely tougher to get your hands on when you don't eat meat. But some foods, like breakfast cereals and some meat substitutes, are fortified with B_{12}. Tempeh also contains some naturally occurring B_{12} because it's fermented; bacteria produce the vitamin. Look for cyanocobalamin, the most absorbable form of the vitamin, in ingredient lists. Your prenatal vitamin should also have a decent amount; you need 2.6 mcg each day. One cup of Total cereal has 6 mcg, so you can knock out this vital nutrient at breakfast.

Gluten-Free

Celiac disease is an autoimmune disorder in which the small intestine becomes inflamed when foods containing the protein gluten are eaten. Gluten is found in wheat, barley, and rye products. If the lining of your small intestine becomes damaged, you can't absorb nutrients properly.

When training to be a dietitian, I learned that celiac sprue—celiac disease, or complete gluten intolerance—was a very rare disorder, and I wouldn't see much of it. The bad news is that the rate of celiac disease is on the rise, with two million Americans currently diagnosed with it.[5] Women are twice as likely as men to get it.[6] But the good news is that the number of delicious gluten-free foods out there is also climbing, and they're a far cry from the paltry array of rice breads and whisper-thin cereals that were available ten years ago.

If you have been diagnosed with celiac disease, it's important to avoid any flare-ups while you're pregnant or breast-feeding. You need to make sure you absorb as many good nutrients from the foods you're eating as you can.

With clearer package labels, it's easier than ever to stay gluten-free. You know you need to avoid anything with wheat, barley, and rye. Kamut—a grain related to wheat—and spelt are also off limits. Oats have generally been on the no-no list for celiacs, not because they contain gluten but because they are usually processed in facilities that also process wheat. But companies like Bob's Red Mill (sold in natural-foods stores and some grocery stores) now have certified gluten-free oats (made in a dedicated wheat-free facility) that are great for making oatmeal or baking. Watch out for the words "hydrolyzed vegetable protein" and "modified food starch" on ingredient labels. Grains on the okay list are corn, rice, quinoa, and buckwheat. You can also find bread and cereal products made with potatoes and soybeans.

For more information and resources related to celiac disease, go to the Food Allergy & Anaphylaxis Network's website at www.foodallergy.org. Another good resource is http://glutenfreegirl.blogspot.com.

Some of my gluten-free favorites:

- **Babycakes.com**. Incredible cookies and cakes.

- **Cravebakery.org**. These brownies are the real deal. Moist, chocolatey, and crave-worthy, and they're made with flaxseed.

- **Mr. Krispers Baked Rice Krisps**. A great replacement for crunchy wheat snacks. Find them in several flavors at Costco and Sam's Club.

- **Bakery On Main's Gluten-Free Granola**. This is the heartiest gluten-free granola I've found yet, with big chunks of dried fruit and puffed corn and rice. Get it at Giant, Wegman's, and Whole Foods.

Feed the Belly Gluten-Free Goodies

Oatmeal Brulée (if made with certified gluten-free oats; page 169)
Morning, Noon, and Night Nut Clusters (page 182)
Citrus-Spiked Rice Pudding (page 165)
Walnut-Maple Syrup Sauce with Vanilla Ice Cream (page 173)
Deconstructed Apple Pie (page 174)
Fruity Booty Salad (page 176)
All the Thirst-Quenching recipes (which start on page 249)

Food Allergies

Until recently, some doctors advised their pregnant patients to stay away from peanut products, dairy, and soy while pregnant and breast-feeding to help prevent food allergies in their unborn children. But a 2008 report from the American Academy of Pediatrics says avoiding these potential allergens during pregnancy is not necessary unless you, your partner, or your child's sibling has a food allergy. The report also found that there's no anti-allergy benefit to waiting longer than six months to introduce solid foods to your infant. The one thing that does seem to help keep your kids allergy-free is to breast-feed them for at least four months, compared with feeding them formula made with cow's milk protein.[7]

If your family has a strong history of peanut, dairy, or soy allergy, your doctor may advise you to avoid eating those products during your pregnancy anyway.

Chapter Nine

Belly Blues— Morning Sickness Survival Guide

Though it'll often hit you at the start of the day, morning sickness can strike any time it damn well pleases—even in the middle of your big sales presentation. It usually pops up around week six, and nearly all women experience it.[1] Some researchers believe the nausea and vomiting that go along with pregnancy evolved as a protective mechanism. It makes sense that your body would guard itself and your growing baby against environmental toxins and microorganisms. Whatever the case, the nausea and sickness that arise during the first trimester are largely thought to be caused by a surge in pregnancy hormones.[2] Several are on the rise during this time, including human chorionic gonadotropin (hCG), cholecystokinin, estrogen, and progesterone. Levels of hCG start to zoom as soon as you become pregnant—it's hCG that turns that pregnancy test pink or blue. It's necessary for successful implantation of the embryo in your uterus, and it's also to blame for making you want to pee every half hour. Good times!

Just like when you have your period and get the double whammy of gastrointestinal upset or diarrhea, a rise in estrogen can cause tummy issues when you're pregnant. And are you tasting something funny? Blame that metallic or bitter taste in your mouth on those surging hormones too. It's a condition called dysgeusia, which some pregnant women get, and it should disappear once your first trimester is over. Eating acidic foods, such as salsa or lemonade, might help get rid of the taste for a little while.[3] Although it's not environmentally friendly, using plastic cutlery instead of metal may also help combat metal mouth.

Some studies have shown that women who begin taking a multivitamin right around conception are less likely to experience nausea and vomiting.[4] It may be due to the B_6 the multivitamin contains, as vitamin B_6 has been shown to help with the symptoms of nausea.[5] However, most doctors don't recommend taking more B_6 than what's already in your prenatal vitamin.

By the time your first trimester is over, your hormone levels even out, and nausea is usually (though not always) replaced by a ravenous appetite.

Easing the Queasies

You can't prevent it, but you can alleviate the symptoms. Here's what you need to get you through your first trimester. Not every food will work for everyone, so experiment to see which does the trick for you. These are generally bland, but comforting, foods. You might even want to keep some of these by your bedside to snack on before getting out of bed in the morning, because nausea is generally worse on an empty stomach. Go ahead…when else would you let yourself get crumbs in bed?

- **Reed's Ginger Beer**. You might also try popsicles made from ginger beer.

- **Saltines**. Barbara's makes Wheatines, which are whole grain and low sodium.

- **Graham crackers**.

- **Dry cereal**.

- **Low-sodium seltzer water with lemon juice**.

- **Gin-Gins**. These great little hard ginger candies from the Ginger People are fantastic because they're individually wrapped. Keep them in your purse and gym bag to combat nausea on the go.

- **Pretzels**. I'm a huge fan of Snyder's Snaps.

- **Corn bread**.

- **Brown rice**.

- **Tapioca or rice pudding**. Kozy Shack makes a nice all-natural one.

- **Applesauce** (make sure to go organic).

- **Preggie Pops and Preggie Pop Drops** (www.threelollies. com). These lollipops and candies are made with small amounts of essential oils including mint, lavender, ginger, lime, etc. Many women say they work like a charm.

- **Lemons**. Suck on a lemon slice, drink some lemonade, or even give fresh lemons a sniff. This citrus fruit seems to help in many ways.

Non-Food Helpers

Keep these in your purse, desk, and car so they're handy whenever you need them.

- **Sea bands or BioBands**. The same wrist bands you can use for motion sickness also seem to work wonders during pregnancy for many women. You can even wear them at night. They work by putting gentle pressure on the P-6 acupressure point on the wrist. Probably not the coolest accessory in the world, but if it works for you, rock it.

- **Mouthwash**. Let's face it: It helps get rid of that awful post-puke taste.

- **Bottle of water**.

- **Mints**.

Belly Tip

Hot and bothered. Heat and humidity can heighten nausea. If you're preggers in the summer, try this refreshing trick: Use popsicle molds (or even ice cube trays) to freeze ginger ale, lemonade, and limeade into icy pops. They're the perfect thing to ease the queasies on a sweltering day, and they're a nice refreshment when you come home from work.

- **Sugar-free gum**.

- **A sachet** filled with pleasant smelling herbs like rosemary, lavender, or mint. Take a whiff when you need relief. You can also just spray facial tissues with herbal sprays (I like the Zum mist ones) and keep them in your purse. I'm also a big fan of individually wrapped wipes from Herban Essentials; in particular, its lavender-infused Yoga Towelette is great for freshening hands and masking unpleasant smells. They're especially handy for quelling queasies on subways, trains, and buses, where funky air often lurks. They sure saved me on many steamy, gross days on the NY Subway.

Belly Tip

Drink up. Sometimes when you're nauseous and sick, it's a chore to choke down water. But it's important to stay hydrated. Once you're dehydrated, try something like Pedialyte Gastrolyte, or diluted fruit juices to rehydrate. These days, you can also get water with added electrolytes, such as SmartWater, which help you hydrate faster. Eating foods rich in potassium—bananas, sweet potatoes, white potatoes, and apricots—will also help you rehydrate.

- **Ziplock baggies**. When there's no place else to turn, these are a lifesaver.

Alternative Treatments

What about acupuncture and acupressure? You may have heard that these Eastern medicine practices—which involve the use of either needles or finger pressure at specific points along the body—can alleviate your nauseous belly. But does it really work? A review study done by the Center for Complementary and Alternative Health Medicine in Women's Health at Columbia University found that acupressure, ginger, and vitamin B$_6$ were the only alternative methods that had a positive effect on nausea and vomiting.[6] Another review study found mixed results for acupuncture.[7]

If you're into experimenting with complementary treatments and your nausea is severe, it may be worth trying acupuncture or acupressure for temporary relief. Just make sure that the practitioner is licensed by your state and comes highly recommended by someone you know.

The Upside of Upchucking

Here's some good news for morning sickness sufferers: Recent research shows that women who experience nausea and vomiting during pregnancy are about 30 percent less likely to develop breast cancer.[8] Plus, it's a sure sign that the embryo is implanted in the uterus. If there's no implantation (which is necessary for a successful pregnancy), you won't experience nausea and vomiting.[9]

Belly Tip

Viva la vinegar. If you're sick of saltines, and nothing else seems like it's helping, take a nip of vinegar. It sounds odd, but it works for a lot of women. I recommend going for a nice aged balsamic over cheaper white vinegar, but see what suits you. Balsamic is great on salads and cooked vegetables, and can even be drizzled on fruit and vanilla ice cream.

Find Your Triggers

Most women experience a heightened sense of smell during pregnancy. Things you used to love the smell and sight of—freshly brewed coffee, grilled meat, and leafy greens, for example—may now make you want to retch. In fact, according to Miriam Erick, MS, RD, CDE, an expert on dealing with severe cases of morning sickness, adverse smells and odors are the most common cause of nausea and vomiting.[10] By making simple changes to your morning routine, or by handing over the kitchen prep or dog-poo pick-up duties to someone else, you may be able to cut down on how often you get sick.

And just like when you're not preggers, getting overheated can make you feel nauseous. You may have loved dining *al fresco* before, but in your knocked-up state, that same sunny patio might pave the way to barf city. Of course, every day will be different, so go by how you feel at the time.

Learn to Graze

Many pregnant women find that the key to avoiding nausea is to eat something every few hours. It certainly worked for me. And slow it down girl: If you used to wolf down meals in ten minutes or less, make an effort to sit down to eat and pace yourself. Not only will eating smaller meals spaced throughout the day help alleviate your nausea, but as your belly grows, you won't be able to pack it quite so full. The same thing is true for liquids. While staying hydrated is important, taking mini sips will make you feel better than gulping. You might find it easier to get your water and other fluids in between meals instead of having them while you eat.

More Than Morning Sickness

Not all women experience morning sickness (lucky them), but some women have a worse time than others. Especially severe morning sickness could be a sign that you're carrying twins: More babies equal extra hormones, and that means more nausea for you.

If you just can't keep anything down, feel ill all the time, and become dehydrated (especially after the first twelve weeks), let your doctor know immediately. You could have hyperemesis gravidarum (HG), a condition that causes extreme nausea, vomiting, and weight loss and sometimes requires hospitalization. The cause is unknown, but it can usually be managed by rest, intravenous fluids, and even acupressure.[11] If you are diagnosed with HG, a great resource is Her Foundation (Hyperemesis Education Foundation; www.hyperemesis.org).

Professional Help

Talk to your doctor if your nausea and vomiting are getting in the way of your daily activities. She may consider giving you B_6 shots or prescribing Zofran (generic: ondansetron), an anti-nausea and vomiting aid.

Chapter Ten

Burps, Farts, Heartburn, Bloating, and Other Good Times

An unfortunate (and oh-so-not-cute) side effect of pregnancy is what happens to your digestive system. Depending on how far along you are, you've probably been experiencing everything from constipation (and possibly hemorrhoids as a result) to uncontrollable gas. One reason: Your system is slowing down, thanks to rising levels of progesterone, and with your ever expanding uterus, there's increasingly little room for food to go and for digestion to take place. Plus, those meddling hormones continue to wreak all sorts of havoc. Here's the gamut of gastrointestinal (GI) disturbances, and how to deal with them.

Heartburn

I always thought that heartburn was something only chili dog-eating truckers got. Boy, was I dumb. Those increased levels of progesterone (which the placenta is churning out in large quantities) in your body cause your esophageal sphincter to become more relaxed. Though it sounds like something that would be close to your tush, the sphincter is actually the little valve that covers up your esophagus and normally keeps all that stomach acid from irritating your throat. When it relaxes, it allows the acid to splash up into your throat, causing heartburn. Heartburn usually shows up during the third trimester, when the baby really starts taking over your body's real estate, and the esophageal valve is physically pushed up. But some women are hit with the burn in their first trimester, like my friend Laura during her second pregnancy. She found relief by laying off the offending foods below (even though they're what she craved most). Some pregnant women get heartburn just from drinking water.[1] Oy vey.

Tips on avoiding the burn:[2]

- Lay off spicy foods.

- Try not to eat a large meal right before going to bed (no later than two hours before bedtime).

- Prop yourself up on pillows while sleeping to keep everything in its proper place.

- Avoid coffee and soda—they often make symptoms worse. The same goes for chocolate.

- If you find that tomato-based sauces, such as marinara, give you heartburn, try going with pesto.

- Avoid taking iron supplements at night. They tend to cause heartburn.

- Milk and other dairy products help coat the throat and stomach and might soothe irritation.

- Antacids, such as Tums, Rolaids, Mylanta, and Maalox, can help, but make sure to check with your doctor before taking them.[3]

Source: American Pregnancy Association Fact Sheet on Heartburn

The Gas We Pass

Oh, joy, as if the bloated ankles (or cankles, as my husband likes to call them), the loss of your waistline, and the inability to stay up past 8:30 weren't enough, you've become a total windbag. Again, blame it on the hormones and the lack of room in your belly. Fine, but at least before you were preggers you usually had the ability to hold in your farts, at least for a while. Now you worry that someone behind you with a lighter might cause significant harm to you or others. Can anything be done to stifle the buildup?

- **Avoid the foods that make it worse**. If cabbage and other cruciferous veggies (Brussels sprouts, broccoli, cauliflower) make your belly expand, you can either avoid them, deal with the consequences (because they're super-healthy), or cook the crunch out of them. Raw veggies of all stripes might cause gas. Beans are pretty much guaranteed to give you gas, no matter what. Soybeans and soy-based foods are part of the gas brigade as well.

- Eating gas-causing foods won't physically hurt you or your baby, but it's sure to come back and bite you in the ass. It can also cause painful cramps. **Taking Beano** when you eat veggies and beans can help cut down on gas. It's generally considered safe to use during pregnancy, but check with your doctor before taking it.[4]

- **Dried and fresh fruits** can make you gassy, but they also help prevent constipation, so it's a classic Catch-22.

- Dairy might also be the culprit. Sometimes pregnancy makes it easier for you to digest milk, yogurt, and other cow's milk products, and sometimes it makes it worse. In general, the good bacteria found in **yogurt and other cultured dairy will help regulate your digestion** and cut down on gas and bloating.

- **Onions and garlic can make you gassy**—especially when they're raw. So stick to cooked and try to keep your portions of super-oniony foods small.

- **Avoid sugar alcohols**. These are a family of reduced-calorie sweeteners used in lots of candy products and they can cause wicked gas. Maltitol, erythritol, sorbitol, mannitol, xylitol, lactitol, and isomalt are all sugar alcohols. Check the label on any food product that says it's made without sugar or no-sugar-added, because it may contain sugar alcohol. If you're super-sensitive to it (I'm one of the lucky ones), you can blow up like the Hindenburg by just eating one serving. Diarrhea is another fun potential side effect of eating sugar alcohols.

- **Almonds and other nuts** can make you gassy. Try sticking to a ¼-cup serving size—about twenty-four almonds or fourteen walnut halves—and see if that helps.

- **Cut the high fiber.** High-fiber cereals are great for packing in fiber, but if you're not used to getting 10 g in a single bowl, they can turn you into a high priestess of cutting the cheese. Try mixing your super-fibrous cereal with another that just has a few grams. Over a month or so, you may be able to work your way up to eating an entire bowl of the high-fiber stuff without the obnoxious effects.

- Gulping air while eating can trap gas, causing burps and farts. So do what Mom told you and **keep your trap shut while you're chewing**. Even though they're fun, avoid drinking through straws, because you'll end up swallowing more air. Chewing gum can also trap gas.

- It all goes back to those **smaller, more frequent meals.** Eating less at a single sitting reduces the chance you'll be plagued with gas.

If all else fails, pull on some comfy sweats and take a walk around the block with the dog. Not only will she not mind if you're a little stinky, but it's also a great way to get things moving…and as my grandmother Selma always said, "It's better out than in."

Constipation and Hemorrhoids

So what more can pesky progesterone do? Lots. Just as it relaxes your esophageal sphincter, it also slows down your digestive system. Food usually gets moved along through the intestines with muscular contractions, but progesterone can slow it down, causing constipation.[5] Becoming dehydrated contributes to constipation, because your large intestine will take whatever water it can get from the food you eat, leaving you with rock-hard excrement that can be very painful to pass. What fun!

Since your system is slowing down and there's added pressure from the weight of your growing uterus, you're probably struggling when you have to poo.[6] Hemorrhoids—well, they're like constipation's evil sidekick. They're actually always around—but when there's additional pressure on your booty canal, the veins in the hemorrhoids can swell and sometimes even burst. Hemorrhoids can develop both internally and externally.

Can you do anything to prevent the 'roids? Absolutely—drink a heck of a lot of water (see recommendation on page 32), avoid straining on the toilet, exercise regularly, and get 28 to 30 g of fiber a day. How can you pack that much into a day?

Try getting several of these fiber-rich foods daily:[7]

1 cup blueberries (fresh or frozen)	4 g
1 cup cooked black beans	15 g
1 cup garbanzo beans (chick peas)	11 g
1 ounce almonds	17 g
1 large apple	5 g
1 large pear	7 g
5 prunes	3 g
6 ounces prune juice	2 g
1 cup Kashi GoLean cereal	10 g
½ cup Kellogg's All-Bran Original	10 g
1 Kellogg's All-Bran Bar	5 g
1 cup cooked whole-wheat pasta	6 g
1 cup cooked brown rice	4 g
½ cup cooked broccoli	3 g
1 cup Brussels sprouts	4 g

1 cup raw carrots	4 g
1 slice Wasa crisp bread	2 g

Sources: www.nal.usda.gov, www.all-bran.com

And yes, there are two types of fiber—soluble and insoluble. The first type, which helps lower cholesterol and blood sugar, is found in oats, peas, beans, apples, citrus fruits, barley, and psyllium. Insoluble fiber is like hay—it doesn't dissolve in water and helps give you a really full feeling, plus it helps you have bowel movements. It's found in whole wheat, bran, nuts, and vegetables. Instead of thinking too much about which type of fiber you're getting, just know that getting both types will help you stay healthy.

Bloating and Swelling

If you're in your seventh month and you can still wear your wedding ring, you're a rock star. Most women are guaranteed to swell up at some point in their pregnancy, especially toward the end. Ankles, calves, hands, and feet are all fair game, but if your face is swelling, you may have preeclampsia. Call your doctor if *both* your face and hands become swollen.[8] Since caffeine is out, you can't turn to that old diuretic staple for help, but there are things you can do to help you feel like less of a water balloon.

Certain foods contain natural diuretic properties. Asparagus is one of them,[9] and it also happens to be rich in folic acid, so it's doubly good for you right now. Celery does the trick, too,[10] so it makes sense to snack on this low-cal cruncher. (Try it with my creamy All-Purpose Veggie Dip on page 232.) Other foods that don't necessarily stimulate the production of urine, but are rich in water, include watermelon (duh), honeydew melon, cantaloupe, and cucumber. It might seem counterintuitive, but drinking water and eating fluid-rich foods can help ease swelling.

Avoiding sodium will also help you beat the bloat. When you've had too much sodium-rich food, your body retains water to try to keep the sodium levels in your body fluids balanced. Drinking more water will help you flush that excess salt out of your system. Eating foods rich in potassium, such as bananas, potatoes, avocado, and cantaloupe, will also help you beat the bloat.

While we do need a certain amount of salt each day, most of us get way too much. Here are some tips for cutting out excess salt:

- **Step away from the shaker**. If you're one of those people who salts her food before she eats, try to kick the habit. Take a couple of bites first, and if it's still bland, add a judicious shake or two.

- **Rinse cycle**. When using canned beans and veggies, rinse them first in a colander. You'll reduce the sodium considerably. As you rinse those beans, you'll also be washing away a lot of their gas-producing polyscaccharides.

- **Get fresh**. Processed foods are high in sodium because it makes food taste good and acts as a natural preservative. If you're eating primarily fresh foods, you're naturally cutting back on sodium (but that's not necessarily true for restaurant food).

Culture Club

Probiotics have been a big buzzword the last few years. These beneficial bacteria—aka live active cultures, like lactobacillus acidophilus—can do you a world of good digestion-wise and also help guard against nasty yeast infections. Yeast infections are more common during pregnancy because vaginal secretions increase in sugar, which provides lots of energy for yeast to feed on.[11] Remember, you can't just pop a Diflucan (a common drug for yeast infections) when you're pregnant, because that medication isn't approved for use by pregnant women. I know, it's a totally gross and uncomfortable situation, but you can fight back against the yeasties with your own army of good bacteria.

What's the magic in the **microbes**? Beneficial bacteria help break down food, making digestion easier. They also help fight bad bacteria in your gut and restore balance to your intestinal microflora. It's kind of like *feng shui* for your belly. Benefits of eating food with probiotics include reduced bloating and indigestion.

Where to get probiotics:

- **Yogurt**. Go for plain and look for sweetened varieties made with less sugar (but not the sugar-free kind)—no more than 20 g of sugar per serving. Often, the kinds with fruit on the bottom have more sugar than the blended style. Greek-style yogurt has become really popular and more widely available in the last few years. It's rich and creamy because it's triple strained; even the fat-free stuff is nice and thick, and it's higher in protein. Use it instead of sour cream in dips and as a topping on tacos and baked potatoes. If you're lactose intolerant, you'll probably be okay with yogurt because the good bacteria help to break down the lactose sugar, leaving less of it for you to digest.

- **Digestive drinks, yogurts, and probiotic smoothies**. These yogurts and drinks, such as Activia, Yo-Plus, and GoodBelly (a great non-dairy option), use specific strains of probiotics to help ease digestive woes and often contain prebiotics as well (read on to find out more about them). However, you usually have to eat or drink them consistently for at least two weeks to see a benefit.

- **Kefir**. This tangy drink is like a cross between buttermilk and yogurt. If you don't like the flavor on its own, try it over cereal or as a base for fruit smoothies.

- **Cottage cheese**. Some brands, such as Nancy's and Kraft's Live-Active, include live active cultures. I know cottage cheese screams "diet plate at the assisted living center!" but it's really quite nice mixed with berries or spread on a piece of hearty toasted bread and topped with tomatoes, salt, and pepper.

- **Enhanced products**. Now that the science behind beneficial bacteria has been confirmed, all sorts of new products have hit the market. There are breakfast cereals with probiotic puffs and flakes (by makers like Kashi and Kraft) and cheese with added cultures. You can even choose great-tasting probiotic chocolate and granola bars from Attune that make it easy to get your fix on the run.

So you know where to get the good bugs, but to make them work even better, make sure to get prebiotics too. Probiotics rely on prebiotics for food, so it's important to get both at the same time for the biggest benefit. Fructan and inulin are prebiotics that are added to several brands of yogurt and probiotic drinks. Prebiotics also occur naturally in foods like artichokes, asparagus, green beans, leeks, onions, barley, and wheat.

You don't need to turn this into a science project and start dousing your green beans in strawberry yogurt, but try to fit in one food with good bacteria each day—preferably one with a prebiotic—and you're likely to see the benefits. Also, keeping your sugar intake under control will help keep your intestinal flora balanced, which adds up to better digestion and fewer yeast infections.

Speaking of Vajayjays...

The dreaded UTI. It's yet another womanly affliction that comes on with a burning sensation when you pee and then launches into a full-scale attack on your urinary tract. Guess what—it's more common when you're preggers. Urinary tract infections, also known as UTIs or bladder infections, are also referred to by doctors as the honeymoon syndrome, because they often crop up after copious amounts of sex. However, there are other causes as well: When you're pregnant, your uterus gets bigger and can get in the way of proper drainage of urine from your bladder. This means that bacteria have a chance to grow, which can lead to an infection.[12]

If you think you have a UTI, call your doctor immediately. If you let it go untreated, it could develop into a kidney infection. Antibiotics usually help you feel better within a day or so. To help prevent an infection, pee when you need to, drink plenty of water daily, and make one glass each day a blend of water and pure cranberry juice (see the Pantry section on page 43 for more on what type to get).[13]

Also, take care of Miss Kitty and dry her daily with the low-heat setting of your hairdryer. Wear breathable cotton panties (there's nothing bacteria like better than a warm, dark, and moist place) and at night, go without knickers.

Chapter Eleven

"Does My Butt Look Fat?" and Other Weighty Questions

An inevitable part of your pregnancy will be weight gain. While some women embrace their new curves and delight in showing them off in stretch jersey, others of us find this "growth" experience to be about as much fun as sitting through an Ultimate Fighting Championship match (at least with that, you get to see some hard-bodied men go after each other in onesies). But even though you're expanding and stretching in places you didn't know you had, rest assured that all this new padding is providing a warm, safe haven for your little one. A bigger ass and boobs are all part of nature's grand plan.

Of course, you might wonder just how much weight is appropriate for you to gain. It all depends on your pre-pregnancy size and how many babies you're carrying. Suggested weight gain during pregnancy is based on guidelines from the National Academy of Sciences' Institute of Medicine. But as with most things in pregnancy, there's an individual element too, and it's something you should discuss with your doctor.

Standard guidelines use body mass index (BMI) to determine how much weight you should gain. You can figure out your BMI by converting your weight in pounds to kilograms (divide by 2.2) and dividing it by your height in meters squared (one inch = 0.0254 meters). Or keep it simple and check out the Centers for Disease Control and Prevention's BMI calculator at http://www.cdc.gov/nccdphp/dnpa/bmi. In 1990, the Institute of Medicine updated its recommendations on maternal weight gain during pregnancy, increasing them from previous guidelines.[1] See the chart below for the current recommended weight-gain guidelines:

Pre-pregnancy weight	Recommended weight gain
Underweight, BMI less than 19.8	28–40 pounds
Normal weight, BMI of 19.8 to 25	25–35 pounds
Overweight, BMI above 25	15–25 pounds
Twins	35–45 pounds, regardless of pre-pregnancy weight

Source: National Academy of Sciences

Basically, Nicole Richie–size women need to gain much more weight to sustain their pregnancies than women who weigh what Star Jones did pre–gastric bypass surgery. Generally, if women don't gain enough during the nine months their baby is growing, there's a greater risk of low birth weight, and therefore, some developmental issues. But new research from Harvard shows that women who gain too much weight during their pregnancies—or even the right amount, according to current guidelines—can have babies that are too large at birth and may tend to be overweight or obese during childhood.[2] A recommended weight range is given because researchers haven't yet found a way to calculate an individual's ideal weight gain. And that's another reason why even though you might gain ten more pounds than your best friend, your babies could still end up at the same weight.

Weight recommendations haven't always been so generous. My mother loves to tell me about how the Army docs (my dad was in the military) made her adhere to a strict limit of 20 pounds for each of her five pregnancies in the 1960s and 1970s. If expectant moms tipped over the 20-pound mark, they were hospitalized and put on a diet. Okay, that's extreme and a bit misogynistic, but the Army was trying to prevent complications during delivery, and now we know that extra weight gain can lead to issues, such as larger babies, preeclampsia, and gestational diabetes. And Mom doesn't hold it against them—those 20 pounds were always pretty easy for her to shed within six weeks of delivery.

It's smart to keep track of your weight pre-conception so your doctor can more accurately pinpoint your target weight gain. You should definitely meet the minimum weight gain suggested, but if you're 5 feet, 2 inches tall and previously weighed 102 pounds, it probably doesn't make sense for you to gain 40 pounds.

Some experts, such as Dr. Emily Oken, MD, MPH, an instructor in the department of ambulatory care and prevention at Harvard University and one of the investigators in the study mentioned above on maternal weight gain, thinks that pregnant women should try to avoid excess weight gain as much as possible. Oken says that a baby's weight at birth can predict what his or her weight will be later on, but a mom's weight gain during pregnancy is an even bigger factor. For the healthiest outcome for both mother and child, Oken suggests that you aim for the low end of the weight range your doctor suggests (for most women, it's about 25 pounds) and make every effort to be physically active (see page 103 for more on exercise).[3] In fact, the Institute of Medicine is presently revising its guidelines; it'll be interesting to see how they change.[4]

Bigger Bellies, Bigger Issues

Let's face it. Women in the United States are getting heavier. The latest government reports tell us that two-thirds of American adults are overweight or obese.[5] Of course, that means that pregnant women are heavier than ever before. Unfortunately, excess weight isn't only linked to heart disease, diabetes, and high blood pressure—it's also tied to complications during pregnancy. Women who start off their pregnancies overweight or obese (a BMI above 25 or 30, respectively) need to keep their weight in check the most. New studies show that overweight or obese women who gain 15 to 25 pounds have a higher risk of having a Cesarean delivery, a larger-than-average baby, and preeclampsia. Women in the study who gained less than 15 pounds had a decreased risk of all these factors.[6]

Other studies show that obese women have longer stays in the maternity ward (likely due to having Cesareans), and also take more medications while pregnant, and require more prenatal testing.[7] Plus, post-delivery deep-vein thrombosis (DVT), which is a condition that causes blood clots to form in deep veins, is more common, which contributes to longer hospitalizations. Of course, more tests and longer hospital stays mean more expenses for you. So vanity and social pressure aside, it makes sense to go into your pregnancy at a healthy weight.

If you're overweight and not pregnant yet, even a weight loss of 10 to 15 pounds will help improve your health. Talk to your doctor about your current weight and whether you should try to lose a little before conceiving. Once you're pregnant, ask her how much she suggests you gain while pregnant. Some doctors advise their obese patients not to gain any weight at all.

For whatever reason, many doctors are reluctant to bring up the issue of weight with their pregnant patients. Maggie Somerall, MD, FACOG, of Premier Women's Care in Birmingham, Alabama, wishes more doctors would advise their patients to keep their weight in check. During her twenty years in practice, she's seen that women who gain too much during their

Belly Tip

Portion pal. Got a craving for rich, velvety ice cream? Put down that pint of Chubby Hubby! You can have the ice cream, but it's a really bad idea to eat it directly from the container. It's easier, of course, but you can't tell how much you've eaten, and if it's a variety with chunks, you'll likely just keep digging for more buried treasure.

Here's the trick—get yourself a really cute bowl or martini glass (I got mine at a secondhand store) that just fits ½ cup of ice cream—the official serving size—and a small, fun spoon. Fill up your bowl and savor each and every bite. That tiny spoon will ensure more bites per cup, and you'll indulge the craving without totally racking up calories. The same is true for other "more-ish" snacks like chips and pretzels—measure out a portion and stick to it.

pregnancies, and keep those pounds on postpartum, have a greater chance of struggling with their weight for the rest of their lives.[8]

If you're a bigger gal, I realize that all of this information is super-depressing. I'm basically telling you that if you're already heavy, you're just going to get heavier when you're preggers, and then stay that way forever. Yes, those are the statistics, but it's not inevitable! While dieting during pregnancy isn't something that most doctors recommend, some recent studies show that for obese women, it may be the smartest move. In a recent study done with pregnant women who were obese and had gestational diabetes, one group was given a diet and exercise plan to follow, and another group was advised to follow dietary recommendations for diabetics. The women who followed the diet and exercise program either lost or maintained their weight throughout their pregnancies, delivered babies that were more likely to be normal sized, and most delivered those babies naturally. However, the sample of women in the study was small—only ninety-six women—so if your BMI is at or above 30, talk to your doctor before starting a diet during your pregnancy.[9]

Of course, you should never take any stimulant- or herbal-based diet supplements while pregnant, so read labels closely. And don't forget to get all the important nutrients detailed in Chapter 2.

Grow, Momma, Grow

Don't bother asking your husband: Yes, your butt does look bigger. BMIs aside, everyone gains weight when they're knocked up. You, me, and even Jessica Alba. You feel like your belly (and hips and tush for that matter) is expanding at a rapid pace, but just how *quickly* are you supposed to be gaining weight? Even though your clothes might be fitting differently and you might start feeling a little frumpy (I know I did), you probably won't gain much weight during your first trimester, and that's perfectly normal.

If you were at a healthy weight before your pregnancy, you should expect a monthly gain of about 1 pound a week during your second and third trimesters. If you were more like Kelly Ripa before you got pregnant, your goal is a little more than a pound a week. And if you're curvier (a BMI of 26 or more), your doctor will only want you to gain 0.66 pounds a week. Of course, each week will be different, so don't become obsessed with the scale. Save that for after the baby comes. *(Kidding!)* Your doctor will monitor your weight at each visit and will let you know if you're on track—or if you need to eat a bit more or cut back on the Häagen-Dazs.

Even if you end up gaining more weight than you were "supposed" to, it's not the end of the world. Plenty of hot moms, such as Kate Hudson, Milla Jovovich, Naomi Watts, and J.Lo all gained somewhere around 50 to 60 pounds during their pregnancies, and all got back to their fab figures pretty quickly. True—they had trainers, dietitians, home gyms, and stylists helping them lose it and look great—but still, it can be done, girl! If you have an active pregnancy, you're more likely to get in shape post-baby. Read on for ideas on getting and staying active for the next nine months.

Pound for pound:

Where does the weight go? Obviously, your boobs, butt, and thighs, but the pounds also go to support structures for the baby you're carrying:[10]

Baby	About 7 ½
Placenta	1 ½
Amniotic fluid	2
Your breasts	2
Your uterus	2
Body fluids	4
Blood	4
Stores of fat, protein, and other nutrients	7
Grand total	30

Source: Planning Your Pregnancy and Birth, Third Edition,
American College of Obstetricians and Gynecologists

Chapter Twelve

Sweating for Two

Whether you hung up your sneakers after that disastrous attempt at softball in ninth grade or you're a certifiable gym bunny, it's good for you and for your baby to get moving. Staying physically active now will help you feel better, manage your stress and anxiety levels, and even help prevent gestational diabetes. Studies have shown that aerobic exercise helps treat mild to moderate depression, which can creep up during pregnancy.[1] It'll also help you get back in shape faster later on.

Need more motivation? Women who exercise during their pregnancies often have an easier and shorter labor, with fewer complications.[2] And regular exercise also helps you keep, uh, regular. Ladies, if that's not an incentive to get your tushes off the couch, I don't know what is.

But if you need another reason, here it is: Children of moms who were active during pregnancy were more likely to exercise themselves. A British study done on eleven- and twelve-year-olds examined the kids' activity levels and compared them to how much their moms walked or swam during pregnancy and when the kids were two years old and under. There's probably not a fitness gene, but parents can set a good example and make fitness a family affair.[3]

If the most intense form of exercise you've done in recent years is shoe shopping, definitely consult your doctor before starting an exercise program. She'll probably tell you to go for it (slowly and easily) as long as you don't have any complications. Look for pregnancy-specific classes at your gym or community center. You'll feel less out of place and will get more out of the workout if you have a qualified instructor guiding you. If you have miscarried before, your doctor may want you to wait until the second trimester to start exercising.

Get started with non-weight-bearing exercises like swimming, water aerobics (great for alleviating lower back pain), and cycling on a stationary bike. Walking is great too. Plus, if you find a walking buddy, you're more likely to stick with it, and you'll be able to fit in more time to socialize, which is also a great mental-health booster.[4]

Remember, the goal of exercising now isn't to get ripped; it's to feel better, stay limber, and prep you for labor. I know that staying active helped me feel more like myself. Once you reach your second trimester, you'll need that 300 extra calories a day, so if you end up burning an additional 250 on the treadmill, make sure to have a bonus snack to replenish what you burned (turn to page 140 for a list of healthy bites).

As always, stay hydrated! Never head out for a walk or start a class without a bottle of water. Try to drink 16 ounces of water *before* you exercise (remember, guzzling these days isn't really an option). During exercise, it's smart to drink 8 ounces of water every twenty minutes, and make sure to drink another 16 when you're done. Yes, this means more trips to the bathroom, but it's important! Dehydration can lead to Braxton-Hicks contractions, and sometimes even real contractions, during the second and third trimesters.[5]

If you stuck to a regular exercise schedule before your pregnancy, you can pretty much keep at it with your doctor's clearance, but there are some things to keep in mind.[6]

As is always the case with exercise—listen to your body. If you feel good, keep going, and if not, back off and take a break.

Tips for safe sweating:

- **It's important not to get overheated**. Avoid exercising in hot, humid weather. If you live in a sultry place like Orlando or New Orleans, you're better off joining a gym in the summer. When you exercise indoors, make sure you're in a well-ventilated space or next to a fan. Even though you may be trying to cover up more these days, make sure your clothes are made of breathable, sweat-wicking fabric.

If you regularly practice bikram or "hot" yoga, it's a smart move to switch over to a regular yoga class. Hot yoga rooms can reach 105°F or hotter and may have humidity levels above 40 percent; I've seen non-pregnant friends pass out from the heat and intensity.[7]

- **Supportive footwear is a must** (no more walking the treadmill in Converse All-Stars!) because your ligaments and tendons are more loosey-goosey during pregnancy thanks to the prevalence of relaxin, a hormone that preps the body for delivery. Unfortunately, loose ligaments can lead to injury, so make sure to replace your shoes regularly (about every five hundred miles of running or walking, or every five months), tie double knots in those laces, and avoid jumping movements. You might be over pronating (rolling the feet inward) more than before your pregnancy because your arches begin flattening out with your increased load. According to Dr. Marlene Reid, spokesperson for the American Podiatric Medical Association and a podiatric surgeon in Westmont, Illinois, heel pain (especially first thing in the morning) is the most common foot-related complaint during pregnancy. This is caused by stretching of the plantar fascia—the band of tissue that connects your heel bone to your toes—which can become swollen and irritated. You might also experience arch pain and ankle swelling.[8] Make sure your sneakers are in good shape, and if you think you're overpronating, buy a shoe that helps correct it. Several companies, including Adidas, make them.

- **Apply sunscreen and wear a hat and sunglasses** if you exercise outside. Your skin is much more sensitive to sunlight because of surging levels of progesterone.[9] As my dermatologist told me, if you think a sunburn is uncomfortable when you're not pregnant, just imagine how you'll feel in your more sensitive state.

- **Avoid or modify one-legged exercises** that require excellent balance. As you get closer to term, the extra 20 to 35 pounds you've gained may throw your balance off.

- **Don't exercise to the point of exhaustion**—you should still be able to carry on a conversation while exercising. And if you feel dizzy or short of breath, stop, rest, and drink some water.[10]

- **Activities with the potential for falling or crashing are off limits**.[11] It's a bummer for super-active types, but it's vital for protecting your bump. Potentially risky sports include skiing, snowboarding, horseback riding, rock climbing, skating (ice or inline skating), cycling on busy roads, skydiving, motorcycling (just because Angelina Jolie did it doesn't mean it's right), contact sports, roller derby, moshing, and any other activity where there's a potential risk of falling. Scuba diving is also a no-no due to the changes in pressure underwater.

- **Warm up and cool down** before and after exercising.[12] Even if you skipped it before, it's super-important now. Warming up with some easy stretches and light walking will help you avoid injury, and decreasing the intensity of the last five to ten minutes of your workout will help your heart rate return to normal.

- **Modify exercises that require you to lay flat on your back** once you reach your second trimester.[13] This position slows blood flow to the uterus. Use an exercise ball for abdominal exercises, and always ask your instructors for modifications. You should also avoid long periods of standing, which are often the norm in body-sculpting classes. But you can sit on a ball or an exercise step and do the exercises from there.

- **Keep on trucking *with* your doctor's approval**. If you were an avid runner before you got pregnant, you can most likely continue running for most of your pregnancy. But research shows that most women find that nausea, discomfort, and fatigue become too great for them to continue running in the third trimester.[14] This doesn't seem to be the case with non-weight-bearing activities, such as swimming, cycling, and using an elliptical machine.

Pilates for Pregnancy

Pilates, with its focus on the core muscles of the back, abdomen, and pelvic floor, is fantastic for pregnancy. It's hard to believe, but you can still work your abs while you're pregnant. If you've ever taken a Pilates class, you undoubtedly heard the instructor tell you to pull your navel toward your spine. With your protruding belly, it might seem unlikely, but the transverse abdominal muscle—which runs horizontally from your hips to your bottom rib—actually lays behind your uterus, so you can still work it by pulling it toward your spine. The transverse works overtime during labor, so it pays to strengthen it during pregnancy. Since this is the muscle that's often referred to as a girdle, learning how to work it can help you find your waistline postpartum.

One issue with traditional Pilates exercises and other abdominal work is that many of the moves are done on the back or the stomach, like "swimming." So it's important to find a class that's geared to pregnant women or taught by someone who knows how to modify the exercises. The most ideal situation is to sign up for a private session with an instructor who can modify an entire workout for you. If you don't belong to a gym that offers classes for the preggers set, order a DVD. There are tons to choose from, such as Sarah Picot's Prenatal Pilates.

Yoga Glow

Yoga is a fantastic form of exercise for expectant moms because the stretching and posture poses help prepare your body for childbirth. If you can embrace the true meditative benefits of yoga, those skills may help keep you calm during the early stages of motherhood, when the kid is working your last nerve and you feel like nothing is going right. Plus, the pelvic and stabilizing exercises that are part of yoga (as well as Pilates) can help you deal with the lower back pain you'll most likely experience at some point in your second and third trimester.[15]

Yoga is also one of the more appealing forms of exercise to ease back into after labor. Look for classes that stick to the safety requirements of the American College of Obstetricians and Gynecologists. Most yoga studios

BUMP-READY ACTIVEWEAR

Since workout gear is so figure-hugging, you'll find that you'll outgrow it long before your regular clothes. You can buy non-maternity clothes that are a size or two bigger before you go for full-on maternity wear. You'll likely use them again when you're breast-feeding and easing back into exercise postpartum. Here are some good options:

Gap Maternity (www.gap.com). You'll find cute, practical, and affordable tops, bottoms, and swimwear. Gap Maternity has really nice *and* sexy maternity panties.

Due Maternity (www.duematernity.com). Due offers fashion-forward swimsuits and bikinis, really nice—but pricey—casual clothes, plus a small but high quality selection of activewear.

A Pea in the Pod (www.apeainthepod.com). This shop has very tasteful, upscale workout gear. You can find some great stuff in the sale rack.

Mimi Maternity (www.mimimaternity.com). The company's selection of activewear is a bit slim, but it offers a lot of great full-coverage bathing suits.

Athleta (www.athleta.com). Nothing special for pregnancy, but Athleta does have a ton of great sports bras. The company also sells fabulous swim dresses that are cute, modest, and have a high ultraviolet protection factor (UPF) rating, which will keep you safer in the sun.

Title 9 (www.titlenine.com). Title 9 doesn't call out products specifically for pregnancy, but it has a very nice selection of sports bras rated on a barbell system. The more barbells a bra has, the more support you'll get.

Motherhood Maternity (www.motherhood.com). These guys have some of the best rated nursing sports bras that can also be used during pregnancy.

Lululemon (www.lululemon.com). Lululemon doesn't make clothes for maternity per se, but the company's great-fitting exercise pants have a high waistband that folds over and stretches with you as you grow. I wore mine throughout my entire pregnancy.

Unbuttoned (www.unbuttonedmaternity.com). This site offers hip mommas a nice collection of curve-hugging activewear and swimsuits from well-known labels, such as Maternal America, Ripe, Prego, and Pure T.

now offer prenatal yoga, so give one a call and ask as many questions as you need to feel comfortable. Ask if the studio needs a signed permission form from your doctor; many do.

If you're currently going to yoga classes or using tapes at home, make sure to avoid inversions (headstand, handstands, etc.) and any deep twists from the waist. Of course, as your belly grows, you don't want to put pressure on your bump with poses that require you to lay on your stomach, like the Cobra. One more tip: Remember to keep breathing throughout the exercises—preferably inhaling and exhaling through your nose—to prevent your muscles from cramping.

Sara Ivanhoe (saraivanhoe.com)[16] is a yoga instructor with almost fifteen years of experience, and she's a generally all-around fantastic person. I asked her to share some rejuvenating yoga poses that are safe for pregnancy and can be done in the privacy of your abode and even in your office (I recommend closing the door). Try them one at a time, or in the sequence listed below. Be sure that you use a sticky yoga mat to help prevent slippage.

Cat/Cow

This one is especially great for alleviating lower back pain (some women swear by it for getting through early labor). Start on all fours, with your wrists directly below your shoulders and your knees right below your hips.

Make sure your spine is neutral (your tush shouldn't be sticking up in the air, and your back shouldn't be bowed). Slowly arch your back and lift your chest and head up towards the sky (cow). Then, tilt the top of your head toward the ground and round your back toward the ceiling (cat). Change the position on each exhale. Repeat five to ten times.

¼ Downward Dog

Instead of the full pose, where you end up looking like an inverted "V," keep your knees bent and position them below your hips. Get there by starting out on all fours. Raise your hips up and back, and position yourself on the balls of your feet. Hold for five breaths and then release back to your hands and knees.

Trikonasana (Triangle Pose)

Start with your legs about a foot and a half apart. Turn your right foot out to the side. Your left foot will be pointing directly in front of you and perpendicular to your right foot. Your hips should be leaning away from your right foot. Reach your right arm out long and then drop your hand down to your shin or ankle (or to a block next to your shin) slowly to maintain your balance. Next, reach your left arm up straight toward the sky, stacking your left shoulder on top of the right one. If you can do it without stumbling, your gaze should follow the left hand. Your left hip should also be stacked on top of the right one. Hold for five breaths and then release and repeat on the left side.

Ustrasana (Camel Pose)

This posture puts gentle pressure on your adrenal glands, which is said to energize you. Instead of doing the full pose, reaching back all the way to your heels, reach back just to your lower back. Start on your knees (if you need some padding, put a folded-up towel or blanket under your knees) with your knees hip-distance apart. Reach both hands behind you and place them on your lower back/buttocks area. Press your hips forward and feel the stretch in your chest. Hold the pose for five breaths and then slowly release and push back to child's pose: arms reaching forward, knees bent beneath you, and belly resting gently on or between your thighs.

Gomukhasana (Cow Face Pose)

Starting on all fours, cross your knees, and sit back on your bottom. Your knees will be crossed in front of you. Reach your left arm up and over your shoulder. At the same time, reach your right arm around your back so your hands meet (don't worry if they can't touch—just use a small towel). Straighten your back so that you get a nice, full stretch for your shoulders and chest. Hold for five breaths. Come back to all fours and cross your legs the opposite way, coming back to a seated position. This time, reach your right arm up and over your shoulder, and reach the left around to meet it.

Paschimottanasana (Seated Forward Bend)

This is a great stretch for your spine and hamstrings. Try it once you've warmed up a bit. Begin seated, with your legs straight out in front of you. Straighten and elongate your spine, exhale, and begin hinging forward from the hips. Your arms should be out in front of you, either resting on the floor, on your shins, or holding your feet. Each time you exhale, try to reach a bit further forward. Avoid rounding your back. Try to think of reaching out beyond your toes instead of simply bending over your legs.

Upavistha Konasana (Seated Wide-Leg Forward Bend)

Begin in the same position as the seated-forward bend. (If your hamstrings are really tight, you may want to place a small rolled-up towel under your tush.) Open your legs as wide as you are comfortable doing. Engage your quadriceps (thigh muscles) and flex your feet. Keeping your spine straight, begin coming forward, using your hands for support. On each exhale, try to stretch forward a little bit more.

Supta Baddha Konasana (Goddess Pose)

Traditionally, this pose is done with your back flat on the floor, but since you can't do that, you need to modify it. Using pillows or bolsters, create a base to lie back on. Recline on the pillows until you're comfortable and then butterfly your legs out. Hold the position for several minutes, breathing deeply.

To come out of the pose, roll over to one side and transition to hands and knees. From your knees, use your hands to help you stand up slowly.

Belly Breathing

If you practice yoga, you're already familiar with *ujjayi* breathing. It's a form of breathing that can help you relax and focus your energy during labor. It can take a bit of practice to master and you might feel a bit silly doing it, but it's good stuff. Here's how to do it: Breathe in through your nose, resting the tip of your tongue on the roof of your mouth. Allow your belly to inflate with oxygen (it may help to rest your hand or a box of tissues on your stomach so you can see and feel it expand). Slowly exhale through your nose, actively pushing out the air from your abdomen. This should make an audible sound, like "hrrr." You can practice your breathing anytime. It's not only good for labor, but for whenever you're feeling stressed. If it doesn't feel good to exhale through your nose, try exhaling through your mouth.

Just Squeeze It

Keeping your pelvic floor strong will help ensure that your vaginal canal can open more easily during childbirth. It will also help you avoid embarrassing issues with urinary incontinence postpartum.

Those notorious Kegel exercises—tightening the inside of your vagina as though you were stopping the flow of urine—will also make sure everything is fully functioning down there after childbirth.[17] Kegels help strengthen your pelvic floor, which is the "hammock" of muscles that holds up your pelvic organs, including your bladder. Do your Kegels on a daily basis—while standing in line at the grocery store, while talking to your mom on the phone, or while shopping for a changing table. The cool thing is that no one can see you doing them. Squeeze the muscles you would use if you were mid-way through peeing and someone opened the door on you. Good. Now hold that for three seconds, and relax for three seconds. Repeat ten to fifteen times a total of three sets a day. Yeah, I know, it's another thing to keep track of, but Kegels only work when you do them consistently. Try setting a daily alarm on your phone to help you remember. Bonus: Kegels can also help keep your vaginal muscles tight, which means that sex will feel better for you. Now, that's an exercise plan we should all want to stick with.

Squat Strengthener[18]

Because labor is usually a marathon, not a sprint, you'll need to build up some endurance in your legs. Sara suggests doing assisted squats to strengthen your glutes, quadriceps, and hamstrings. Luckily, you can do this exercise in any room that has a door. Simply shut the door securely, grab the doorknob with both hands, place your feet hip-distance apart, and ease back into a squat. Hold for a count of five and repeat five times. You can build up to ten sets of ten counts each.

Don't Overdo It

Stop exercising and contact your doctor immediately if you have any of the following symptoms:[19]

- Vaginal bleeding.

- Dizziness or feeling faint.

- Increased shortness of breath.

- Chest pain.

- Headache.

- Muscle weakness.

- Calf pain or swelling.

- Uterine contractions.

- Decreased fetal movement.

- Fluid leaking from the vagina.

Chapter Thirteen

When Things Get a Little Complicated

Gestational Diabetes, Preeclampsia, Pregnancy-Induced Hypertension (PIH), and Twins!

Gestational Diabetes

So you've been eating a steady diet of Ding-Dongs and angel-hair pasta, and now your doctor tells you you've got gestational diabetes mellitus (GDM). Or maybe you've been following a completely whole-food diet and limiting portions, but your blood glucose was still high at your last exam. Let's face it, even glam goddesses like Angelina Jolie and Salma Hayek (reportedly) developed GDM during their pregnancies.

Either way, don't beat yourself up about it. Between 3 and 5 percent of all pregnant women develop GDM, and rates are on the rise, likely because more women are obese and/or older when they become pregnant. Certain ethnic groups are at greater risk for GDM.[1] Rates are on the rise for diabetes in general (both Type 1 and Type 2) for women of all ages and ethnicities.[2]

So why does diabetes develop when you're pregnant? Those same hormones that the placenta produces to maintain your pregnancy can also interfere with insulin's role in bringing glucose to your body's cells. Even though your body is making more insulin than it did before you were pregnant, sometimes it's not enough to handle all the sugar in your blood, and that creates insulin resistance. If your doctor tells you your blood glucose level is borderline high, a few dietary changes may do the trick. Once my sister dropped her bag-of-gummy bears-a-day-habit, her blood sugar level returned to normal. When my friend Tanya gave up her sugar-smacked Kool-Aid, she too was able to avoid GDM.

You're at greater risk for GDM if you fit into the following categories, but keep in mind that many women who don't have any of these risk factors end up developing gestational diabetes:[3]

- You're of African-American, Asian, Latino, Native-American, Pacific Islander, or South Asian descent.

- You're overweight or obese.

- You're not physically active.

- You have high blood pressure.

- You have high cholesterol (more than 200 total).

- You're carrying multiples.

- You've previously been diagnosed with GDM.

- You have a family history of diabetes.

- You have polycystic ovary syndrome (PCOS).

- You have a history of cardiovascular disease.

- You're age thirty-five or older.

Side Effects/Dangers of Having GDM

Often, a woman won't know she has GDM because she doesn't have any symptoms. But blurred vision, fatigue, frequent infections (like bladder infections), increased urination and thirst, or weight loss despite an increase in appetite are common side effects. Of course, several of these symptoms go hand in hand with pregnancy, so it can be tough to pick up on a change. Your doctor should screen you for GDM between twenty-four and twenty-eight weeks, because a surge in pregnancy hormones during that period can cause insulin resistance. If you have risk factors for GDM, the American

College of Obstetrics and Gynecology says you should get tested at your first prenatal visit.[4]

What to Expect

If you are diagnosed with GDM, your doctor will advise you to control your blood glucose with diet. But God bless them, doctors aren't always the most gifted people for communicating nutrition and diet advice. Ask your doctor to refer you to a registered dietitian (RD) who will provide you with specific dietary guidelines. You can find an RD in your area at www.eatright.org.

Here are some basics:

- If you've followed the advice in this book, you're probably already eating **small, frequent meals**. To better manage your blood sugar, you need to make meals smaller and more frequent to help keep things stable.

- Make an effort to eat a combo of **healthy fats, whole grain and high-fiber carbohydrates, and lean protein** at each meal. An ideal meal would be a spinach salad with grilled chicken and avocado, or black-bean soup with a small whole-grain roll.

- Add **daily moderate exercise** to your schedule. Physical activity helps lower your blood glucose levels. Talk to your doctor about how much exercise you should aim for.

- Post-pregnancy, keep up a **healthy diet and regular exercise**. Many women with gestational diabetes develop full-on diabetes within five to ten years after delivery.

Your doctor should monitor your blood glucose level at each appointment for the rest of your pregnancy, and she may ask you to check it daily at home with a glucose monitor as well. If dietary modifications aren't working well enough to control your blood sugar, you may need to start taking insulin. Also, your doctor may perform an ultrasound and a non-stress test between weeks thirty-eight and forty-two (if you're overdue). The non-stress test reads your baby's heart rate as he's moving in your belly.[5] These tests can be performed as early as the beginning of the third trimester.

Preeclampsia (Also Known as Toxemia and Pregnancy-Induced Hypertension)

Preeclampsia is pregnancy-induced high blood pressure, coupled with the presence of protein in your urine. The cause of preeclampsia isn't known, but researchers think it might be linked to poor nutrition, a high amount of body fat, and possibly insufficient blood flow to the uterus. If you already have high blood pressure, have a family history of preeclampsia, are clinically obese, are carrying more than one baby, are having your first baby, or have a history of diabetes, lupus, kidney disease, or rheumatoid arthritis, you're also at risk. Sounds pretty unavoidable, right? Well, one thing you can do is to make sure you're getting enough vitamin D. Inadequate vitamin D levels in early pregnancy have been linked to a fivefold increase in the risk of preeclampsia.[6] See page 23 for more on vitamin D.

There's been some promising preeclampsia research on the benefits of lycopene, the antioxidant found in foods like tomatoes (especially cooked tomato products), watermelon, apricots, and pink grapefruit. A study done in New Delhi, India, on women in their first pregnancy found that women who were given lycopene from a tomato extract were about 50 percent less likely to develop preeclampsia.[7] Whether this would hold true for women eating a typical Western diet is unclear, but it can't hurt to enjoy lycopene-rich foods like pasta sauce, watermelon juice, and gazpacho (turn to page 243 for my Peasant-Style Gazpacho).

You're also more susceptible if you're thirty-five or over.[8] Since the percentage of women over thirty-five having babies is on the rise, so is preeclampsia. You're in good company—even thin *Desperate Housewives* star Marcia Cross developed the condition when she was preggers with her twins. She was placed on bed rest for two months.[9]

Body mass index (BMI) also appears to play a role in whether you'll develop preeclampsia. In a study that followed more than one thousand pregnant women, researchers found that those with a pre-pregnancy BMI of 30 (clinically obese) had three times the risk of preeclampsia. And skinny minnies with BMIs of 17 and 19 before pregnancy had a reduced risk of 57 percent and 33 percent, respectively.

If you have risk factors for preeclampsia, especially high blood pressure or kidney disease, you'll want to see your doctor regularly so she can note any fluctuations in your blood pressure or weight.

Preeclampsia causes swelling of the hands and face, rapid weight gain, headaches, and blurred vision. If you develop this condition, your doctor will monitor you closely and check your blood pressure, urine (for protein), and weight at each visit. Your visits will likely become more frequent. If your blood pressure remains high, you might be placed on bed rest.[10]

Twins

So you've got a double blessing coming your way? *Mazel tov!* You probably have twice as much on your mind as most moms to be, not to mention anxiety over how you're going to pay for all the stuff that goes with your matching bundles of joy, like that ridiculously expensive double baby jogger. Although twin pregnancies don't necessarily come with any more complications than singles, you'll be working overtime to make sure you're taking in all the nutrients your developing duo need.

Twin births are still special, but they're not as rare as they used to be. The number of twin births increased 42 percent between 1980 and 1997, mainly in women thirty and older. The rate of twins increases an astronomical 1,000 percent for women forty-four to forty-nine.[11] The fact that moms of "advanced maternal age" are having a ton of twins isn't just due to fertility treatments that often result in multiple births; it's also because of the way women thirty-five and over ovulate. As women age, the level of follicle-stimulating hormone (FSH) rises, and that can lead to double ovulation.[12] These twins are fraternal instead of identical, because they come from separate eggs. So even though the number of eggs you have after thirty-five is on the decline, the probability that you'll be buying a double stroller and matching onesies increases dramatically.[13]

If you've got two buns, your doctor will usually want you to gain more weight to ensure your babies are big enough at birth. (J.Lo certainly took her doctor's advice to heart, packing on 50 pounds during her pregnancy and glowing all the way.)

Because you need even more nutrients and calories than ladies carrying just one bun in the oven, you'll need to plan for some serious mini-meals. You might need four or five snacks a day instead of three. Instead of eating 250 calories at a time, try mini snacks of just 100 to 150 calories or so. It could be one cheese stick, four whole-grain crackers, or even half an apple and 2 teaspoons of peanut butter (turn to page 140 for some Momma Munchies that average around 100 to 150 calories).

Your doctor may also prescribe more iron and folic acid supplements in addition to what you're getting in your regular prenatal vitamin. If you're taking more iron, you'll be more likely to suffer from constipation, so drinking plenty of fluids and getting enough fiber is super-important.

Phenylketonuria (PKU)

This is an inherited disorder that causes a buildup of the amino acid phenylalanine because the body can't break it down. Babies are screened for PKU at birth, so adults who have it have been dealing with it their entire lives. Women with phenylketonuria must follow a special low-protein diet both before and during pregnancy to make sure their levels of phenylalanine don't reach dangerous levels. People with PKU need to also steer clear of anything sweetened with aspartame (NutraSweet). High levels of the amino acid can cause mental retardation and other developmental problems in babies.[14]

Chapter Fourteen

Germ Patrol

How to Make Your Kitchen, Fridge, and Desk a No-Bacteria Zone

I know you have enough to worry about already. You're trying to pack in all the nutrients you need for that growing baby while not gaining too much weight or eating the wrong type of cheese in the process. But if you take a few extra steps, you'll be much safer, and therefore happier, in the long run. You don't want a nasty foodborne illness to sideline you or potentially harm your baby. These days, we're not just dining out or preparing meals in our kitchen, we're also eating at our desks and in our cars. Here's what you need to know to keep all the places you eat clean and bacteria-free.

Banish Bacteria and Viruses

Before you were pregnant, you might have gotten away with eating last Thursday's leftover Thai food for lunch on Monday, or enjoying a bloody rare steak. But now that you're pregnant, your body is more susceptible to foodborne illness and bacteria that like to hang out in food, such as *Salmonella* and *Listeria*. Foodborne bacteria can cross the placenta, and since your baby doesn't have a developed immune system, she's especially at risk.[1]

Some of the symptoms of foodborne illness are similar to those of pregnancy—namely, nausea and vomiting—so it's good to become familiar with the causes so you can seek treatment quickly if you do pick something up. You can't live in a bubble (though sometimes my husband wished I could when we were expecting) or live off hermetically sealed foods, so the best thing to do is play it safe. It's not a whole lot of fun reading about all the stuff that can potentially make you or your unborn baby sick, so let's get it out of the way. Here are the basics:

Campylobacter

It might not sound familiar, but *Campylobacter jejuni* is the number one bacterial cause of diarrhea in the United States.[2] It can be found in raw milk, untreated water, raw and undercooked meat, poultry, or shellfish. This bacteria can cause diarrhea (sometimes even the bloody variety), stomach cramps, fever, muscle pain, headache, and nausea. *Campylobacter* can make you sick two to five days after eating the contaminated food. Even though it's the number one cause of diarrhea, it's pretty easy to avoid as long as you don't eat any raw protein-based foods or drink contaminated water. That's why it's a better idea to take a babymoon in Hawaii or Key West instead of Guatemala or Mumbai.

Clostridium Botulinum

Yes, this is the bacterium that causes botulism, and some of you may even have used a variation of it to smooth your brow. *Clostridium botulinum* produces a toxin that causes muscle paralysis. The biggest offenders for harboring *C. botulinum* are homemade canned and prepared foods that are low in acid.[3] Even though you love Aunt Sally's pickled green beans and have eaten them for years, it's time to regift them to a non-pregnant friend. And I wouldn't recommend taking on any home canning projects right now unless you're a pro. At the store, skip any canned items that are dented.

Early signs of botulism appear four to thirty-six hours after ingesting the bacteria; they include blurred vision and dry mouth, followed by nausea and vomiting. Because the infection can be fatal, it's important to seek treatment immediately if you suspect you've eaten a contaminated food. One more word on botulism: Never give your baby honey (or any foods sweetened with honey) until she's older than a year. Honey can contain *botulinum* spores, which can then multiply in an infant's digestive tract.

Clostridium Perfringens

This bacteria is the bane of church socials and cookouts. *Clostridium perfringens* also produces spores that can grow on meat, meat products, and gravy that are undercooked or left out at room temperature for too long. It can cause abdominal pain, diarrhea, and sometimes nausea and vomiting. The tricky thing with *C. perfringens* is that it sneaks up on you, taking as long as eight to twelve hours to make you sick.[4] You can help avoid it by not eating at places like state fairs and amusement parks, especially during warm weather. When you picnic, make sure to keep cold foods cold and hot foods hot by using an insulated picnic basket or tote. Be sure to eat up before two hours have gone by.

E. Coli

Escherichia coli has developed quite a reputation for making large numbers of people sick at one time, usually because of outbreaks at restaurants or, more recently, due to particular foods, such as bagged spinach. Not all *E. coli* strains make people sick, but 0157:H7 is especially nasty.[5] This particular strain of the bacteria causes diarrhea—often with bloody stools—and can lead to kidney failure and even death in young children. In addition to uncooked produce and raw hamburger meat, the bacterium is also found in raw milk, unpasteurized juice, and contaminated water.

Avoid *E. coli* contamination by cooking all meat thoroughly and using a meat thermometer to test for doneness (see below for more on that). What about bagged lettuce and spinach? The infamous 2006 outbreak originated from one area in the Salinas Valley in California that supplies more than half of the salad greens we eat in this country.[6] So many people got sick because we were all eating lettuce and spinach from the same source. If we were all eating local produce, it wouldn't have happened. But I digress.

You may have gone back to washing and trimming your own salad greens instead of buying the prewashed variety, and that's great. It's also fine if you stuck with the prewashed greens. One thing you don't want to do is *rewash* the stuff that's already been washed. Why? It's already been washed in a mixture of water and chlorine (yup—even the organic stuff), which is more than you can do at home. If you choose to wash your own spinach, lettuce, arugula, etc., remove the outer leaves first, and then wash them in a salad spinner device. After washing, clean your sink thoroughly with an antibacterial spray. After all, if there are any bacteria present on the greens, they're going to get spread all over your sink when you wash them. (For more on keeping your sink safe, turn to page 130.) I'm not trying to scare you away from eating your leafy greens; I'm just trying to help you weigh your options.

Salmonella

Make sure the eggs you use have clean, uncracked shells. But even if they're pristine, eggs can still carry *Salmonella*, a foodborne bacteria that causes salmonellosis—an infection that triggers diarrhea, abdominal cramps, and fever. Symptoms start within eight to seventy-two hours after the contaminated food is eaten.[7] In most people, salmonellosis goes away after a few miserable days, but for people with compromised immune systems like the elderly, young kids, cancer patients, and yes—pregnant women—it can be life-threatening.

You probably already knew that eggs can carry *Salmonella* on their shells, but there are other ways to get the bacteria, too. Uncooked (and undercooked) chicken and meat can carry and spread it to other foods (such as lettuce), which is why it's so important to clean up those chicken juices on the counter and wash your hands thoroughly after handling any raw meat.

As gross as it sounds, some pets can also harbor the bacteria. If you or your kid has a reptile, avoid touching its feces and always wash your hands after handling the snake, lizard, etc. Even if the animal is healthy, it can still carry the bacteria—sorry, all you iguana lovers out there. Baby chicks and ducklings can carry *Salmonella* too.

Trust me, I've heard horror stories about getting sick from *Salmonella,* and you don't want to get it. Follow these tips and you'll stay safe:[8]

- **Keep eggs refrigerated**. Fresh eggs will keep for four to five weeks after you buy them if they're kept in the refrigerator in their original container.

- **Cook eggs completely**, until the yolk and white are firm. Skip sunny-side-up, poached, and soft-boiled eggs.

- Hard-cooked eggs can be kept **in the refrigerator for up to one week**. Ditch them after that.

- **Thoroughly cook foods containing eggs**, such as bread pudding, frittatas, and stratas. Use a meat thermometer to make sure they reach 160°F.

- **Avoid homemade buttercream** or meringue-style icings—the eggs aren't thoroughly cooked.

- It's tempting, but **don't lick the spatula** after mixing up cookie, brownie, or cake batter or homemade frosting.

Listeriosis

We've touched on this one before, but if you've been reading any of the handouts your doctor has given you, you've probably come across the term *Listeria monocytogenes*, the bacterium that causes the foodborne illness listeriosis. Listeriosis causes fever, headache, fatigue, muscle aches, nausea, and vomiting. But the reason why *Listeria* is such an issue for pregnant women is that even if it doesn't make you feel sick, you can still pass it along to your baby. Plus, unlike other bacteria that can't multiply under refrigeration, *Listeria* can thrive at 33°F.

During the first trimester, listeriosis can cause miscarriage, and during the third trimester, your own health is more at risk. This illness can also lead to premature labor, the delivery of a low-birth-weight infant, or infant death. Fetuses who suffer a late infection may develop a wide range of health problems, including mental retardation, paralysis, seizures, blindness, or impairments of the brain, heart, or kidney.[9]

Okay, we're obviously not going to let this happen. The foods that cause the biggest risk of listeriosis are refrigerated, ready-to-eat foods like meat, poultry, seafood, and unpasteurized milk and products made with unpasteurized milk. I'm talking about foods like hot dogs, sliced lunch meats, pâtés, seafood salad, coleslaw, lettuce, and soft cheeses like queso fresco (a fresh, soft Mexican cheese).[10] You can safely eat hot dogs and lunch meats, but they must be heated to a steamy 165°F. Since steaming bologna isn't that appealing and not particularly healthy to begin with, I suggest skipping those processed meats entirely.

Norovirus

This is the one food-related illness that isn't caused by a bacteria; instead, it's caused by a virus. There have been several made-for-TV movie-type outbreaks on cruise ships in the past few years. Other locations that are prime spots for norovirus are nursing homes, hospitals, schools, summer camps, and even large family dinners. Basically, an outbreak can occur any place where one sick food handler could contaminate several people's meals.

Belly Tip

Wiener woes.
Microwaving hot dogs might seem like the way to go for safety, but since microwaves can heat unevenly, it's not a good idea. Boiling is a safer bet, but you'll still want to make sure the temp gets up to 165°F.

The virus is spread through either eating food that's been handled by someone with the virus or direct human contact. It causes gastroenteritis (stomach flu) symptoms, including projectile vomiting, within twenty-four to forty-eight hours after eating or drinking a contaminated food or beverage.[11] Foods commonly affected include raw oysters, shellfish, coleslaw, salads, baked goods, frosting, contaminated water, and ice cubes made from contaminated water.

What can you do to avoid it other than stay as far away from the Love Boat as possible? I'd also skip big community food fairs and chicken dinners, because the food is often being handled by people with no food safety training and may end up hanging out for too long at unsafe temperatures. If you know people who are currently infected with the virus, stay away from them until their symptoms have completely cleared up. If you happen to be taking care of someone infected with the virus, find a way to get him or her cared for by someone else while they are sick. This is disgusting, but their vomit and feces are highly contagious, and everything that these substances get on, including diapers, sheets, towels, and furniture, can pass along the virus to you.

The reason why norovirus is such a concern for pregnant women is that you can easily become dehydrated from it, and you're already more susceptible to getting dehydrated when you're pregnant.[12]

Vibrio

This one's short and sweet: If you don't eat raw shellfish, you won't get *Vibrio vulnificus.* Vibrio shows up during warm summer months in oysters and other seafood.[13]

If you're healthy and not pregnant, it won't do much more than give you a bad case of the runs. In addition to eating food that's contaminated with *Vibrio*, you can also get it if you have an open wound and are in the ocean where there's a high concentration of the bacteria. Symptoms of contamination are sudden chills, fever, nausea, and vomiting. Some people even get blistery sores on their legs.

Belly Tip

Get bratty. If you do get a case of the runs, don't take Pepto-Bismol or Imodium; neither drug has been tested on pregnant women. Instead, you can follow the BRAT diet when you have diarrhea: **b**ananas, **r**ice, **a**pplesauce, and **t**oast. Also, rather than going with whole grains on the BRAT diet, stick to white rice and white bread, because they're low in fiber. All of these foods will help slow the flow and are easy on an upset stomach.

Kitchen Smarts

Even if you don't do much more in your kitchen than heat things up and dump bagged salad into a bowl, it's still important to play it safe. To make sure *Listeria*, *Salmonella, E. coli*, and other bacteria don't find their way into your food, take these steps. Shelley Feist, the executive director of the Partnership for Food Safety Education (PFSE), recommends following the tried and true practices of clean, separate, cook, and chill.

Clean[14]

Wash your hands! It all goes back to what your mom drilled into you as a kid. It's some of the best advice she ever doled out, because it does a world of good. Wash them with warm, soapy water for twenty seconds before and after touching food, and especially after handling raw meat. Dry your hands with either paper towels or a clean cloth towel.

Wash all produce, including those with a skin or rind, like oranges and melons. They may have bacteria on the outside, and when you slice into them, you could be giving those bugs a free ride into the part of the fruit that you're going to eat.

Don't re-wash packaged meat, like chicken breasts. If you cook the meat properly, you'll kill any bacteria that exist. The only thing you'll accomplish by washing it is spreading more bacteria around your sink and work space.

Cutting boards, countertops, and knives need to be washed with hot soapy water after preparing each food. That's why I recommend owning several plastic cutting boards.

Use paper towels to clean up spills. If you use cloth towels, make sure to wash them often in the hot cycle of your washing machine.

The PFSE suggests sanitizing countertops with a solution of 1 tablespoon liquid chlorine bleach (avoid inhaling the fumes) in 1 gallon of water. Let the solution stand on the surfaces for a few minutes; then air dry or pat dry with clean paper towels. It's a super-cheap way to clean, but for its convenience and because I don't want to inhale bleach fumes, I like Clorox Anywhere Hard Surface daily sanitizing spray. It's basically just watered-down bleach in a spray bottle, but if you're not up to mixing it yourself, it's the easy way to keep things clean. Always wear gloves when you're handling chemicals to prevent their absorption into your skin.

Want a greener alternative? White vinegar also kills most bacteria.[15] And companies like Shaklee, Seventh Generation, and Green Works (made by Clorox) make some really effective cleansers that are safer for the environment.

Separate[16]

Use one cutting board for raw vegetables and fruit and a separate one for raw meat, poultry, and seafood. Clean knives with hot, soapy water in between cutting meat and raw vegetables. When you bring your groceries home from the store, place your fresh meats, poultry, and seafood on the bottom shelf of the refrigerator so they can't leak juices (*eww*) onto other foods.

What's the best board?

My mom was upset when I made her throw out her old, cracked wooden cutting board. The problem is that porous and cracked surfaces are too hard to keep clean, and little nooks and crannies are great breeding grounds for bacteria.

- The smartest thing to do is choose boards made from plastic, heatproof ceramic (I like the ones from Epicurean), marble, or tempered glass. Get two different colors and use one for fruits and vegetables and the other for meat, poultry, and seafood. It will help prevent you from cross contaminating things that are going to be eaten raw, like fruit and salad ingredients.

- Run your cutting boards through the dishwasher, or wash them with hot soapy water. To thoroughly sanitize them, wash your boards with a solution of 1 tablespoon of bleach in 1 gallon of water.

- If your board has gotten nicked or cracked, it's time to replace it.

- You can still use your nice wooden boards, but save them for slicing bread or cheese.

Cook[17]

Cook all meat completely. Your days of beef carpaccio are over, my friend. Beef should reach an internal temperature of 160°F, and chicken and other poultry should be at least 165°F, but you might want to cook it longer to get rid of the pinkness completely. Pork, veal, and lamb must reach 160°F. Fish should be 145°F, and the flesh should be opaque and flake easily.

Eggs should be cooked until the yolks and whites are both firm. Egg dishes, like frittatas and casseroles, need to reach 160°F.

Use an instant-read meat thermometer to test the temperature by sticking the probe into the thickest part of the meat and avoiding the bone. You can find these gadgets at cooking stores and bed-and-bath stores for about $15 or less. If you've poked a piece of meat once and the temp isn't high enough yet, remember to wash the thermometer probe before sticking it back into the meat. Yeah, it's a lot to remember, but once you start doing it on a regular basis, it'll become old hat.

Chill[18]

Avoid the "danger zone" of 40°F to 140°F. Make sure your fridge is at 40°F or below by using an appliance thermometer (pick up a cheap one at the hardware store).

- Refrigerate all perishable groceries as soon as you bring them home from the store. The door of your fridge seems like the perfect place to put your milk and juices, but since that area is often not as cold as the main part of your fridge, use it for beverages that don't need to be kept quite so cold, like water. Use the top shelf of your fridge for milk and juice.

- Put all leftovers and takeout foods in the fridge within two hours.

- Keep leftovers for no more than three days and make sure to heat them thoroughly before eating. Microwave ovens often heat unevenly, so check to ensure your food is steaming hot inside before digging in.

- Scan the fridge weekly and chuck anything that's past its date.

- For more information on keeping your food safe, go to www. befoodsafe.org.

The Sink

Believe it or not, your kitchen sink is one of the most bacteria-ridden places in your home. You rinse a lot of different things in there, and bacteria can stick and multiply. Keep your sink area clean and safe by taking the following steps:

- **Use a disinfecting spray** in and around your sink each time you rinse off fresh produce, such as lettuce or grapes.

- Once a week, **give the sink a good scrubbing** (or better yet, have someone else do it). Rinse it with hot water.

- Any time you use cleaning products, **make sure the area is well ventilated** and that you're wearing gloves. Open a window or turn on a fan.

- **Sanitize kitchen sponges** regularly by running them through the dishwasher, which kills about 99 percent of bacteria. Replace them every month.

- **Always wash your hands** after handling raw meat, produce, pets, diapers, or that germy kitchen sponge. The key is to wash with warm water and soap (it doesn't have to be antibacterial) for at least twenty seconds—it takes that long to make sure all the bacteria are annihilated. Make sure you're soaping up long enough by singing "Happy Birthday" or the first refrain of "Like a Virgin."

Dining Out

Since most of us dine out an average of 4.2 times a week, that means that we're preparing less of our own food.[19] That's great for your stress level and aching feet, but if you're not cooking, you can't control how your food is prepared or what goes into it. Before you get too freaked out (like I did), remember that food-service establishments must adhere to food safety guidelines and are subject to routine inspections. Still, if you walk into a place and get the vibe that it's just not up to cleanliness standards, trust your gut and go someplace else.

What else can you do? Shelley Feist from PFSE recommends that you always order your food thoroughly cooked through. If your food arrives lukewarm or still pink in the middle, send it back. No one's going to mess with you—you're preggers. You already know not to order raw seafood or undercooked egg dishes, but remember that many recipes are made with raw eggs. Skip Caesar salads (or ask if they use pasteurized eggs instead of regular eggs), custards, homemade ice cream, eggnog, and sauces made with raw eggs, like hollandaise. Sadly, buttercream icing (unless it's made with pasteurized eggs) is off limits too.

Belly Tip

Bad kitty. If you've got a cat in the house, start looking for someone else to clean out the litter box. Toxoplasma is a parasite that causes *toxoplasmosis*—an infection that causes flu-like symptoms and can lead to miscarriage in pregnant women. Eating raw and undercooked meat is one route of infection, and direct contact with cat poo is another way.[20] It's better to get someone else to clean out that nasty mess on a daily basis, but if you have to do it yourself, make sure to wear disposable gloves and avoid inhaling dust from the litter. Soil can also harbor the parasite, so make sure to wear gloves when gardening. One more thing: If your kids have a sandbox, cover it when it's not being used to prevent neighborhood cats from taking a dump in it.

If you bring a doggie bag home, make sure it gets into the fridge within two hours (one hour if it's 90°F or hotter outside). If you plan to stroll home leisurely or meet friends after dinner, it's probably smart to leave your leftovers on your plate.

Your Desk

It doesn't matter if you work from home or you're a corporate queen, eating at your desk has become the norm these days. Our perma-plugged-in society means that we're trying to get more done in less time. In fact, an American Dietetic Association study revealed that 75 percent of us eat at our desks regularly.[21] I'd rather see you use your lunch break for a quick walk or a relaxing manicure, but I totally understand that sometimes those deadlines make you a slave to your desk. With all those desk-side sandwiches, salads, lattes, and scones come crumbs, grease, and, yes, bacteria, too. One study that swabbed desks to show what type of bacteria were present on the surfaces found they contained *E. coli*, *Streptococcus*, *Salmonella*, and *Staphylococcus aureas* (staph).

Belly Tip

Say no to foam. Though plenty of restaurants are going with more eco-friendly options these days, many of them still send home leftovers in Styrofoam containers. They're not great for the environment, and they're also not good for your health. Transfer your leftovers to a ceramic plate or glass dish before heating them up in the microwave. Styrofoam is not made to withstand the high temperatures microwaves can produce, and these containers may break down and leach chemicals into your food. The same thing goes for soft plastic containers, like margarine tubs and yogurt cups—don't use these plastics for microwaving your food. Make sure all your plastics say "microwave-safe" or have a microwave-safe symbol on the bottom—that means they can withstand the heat without leaching harmful chemicals.

Unfortunately, ladies, we're the worst offenders. Even if our offices look neater, they're actually teeming with more germs. A study done by the University of Arizona and The Clorox Company found that women's desks harbor seven times more bacteria than men's.[22] That's because we tend to stash more snacks in desk drawers, our purses are covered in bacteria, and we gab more, getting our phones covered with those little nasties.

I'm not telling you to not eat at your desk (I mean, when else are you going to work on your baby registry?) or wear white gloves when using the phone. Just keep it clean, girl. Keep a canister of disinfecting surface wipes, which clean up to 99.9 percent of bacteria, in your desk drawer. Make sure they're alcohol-based, because alcohol breaks down the proteins in bacteria, killing them. Wipe down surfaces each time you finish eating and let them air dry.

Clean your phone, keyboard, and mouse while you're at it, as those are big-time germ party spots. And remember, you need to actually get those surfaces *wet* to do any good. Can't do it daily? Give everything a wipe down before you leave for the weekend. Studies show that people who use disinfectants in their offices have less than a quarter of the amount of bugs in their workspace than people who don't.

You might also want to get an easy-to-clean mat to set your lunch on. You know, the type they make for kids. Only now they come in much cooler designs, like the silicone ones from Modern-Twist (www.modern-twist.com).

Your Purse

It turns my stomach just to think about it, but when you set down that Marc Jacobs purse on a bathroom or restaurant floor, it can pick up a whole host of bacteria, like *Salmonella*, *E. coli*, and even superbad *Staphylococcus*.[23] Now that you're eating every few hours and your purse has turned into your second pantry, there are likely to be more crumbs and such in your bag. What's a girl to do?

Skip the suede, because it's tougher to clean than leather or vinyl. Canvas and neoprene totes (like the ones made by Built) are great carryalls because they can be thrown into the washing machine. For leather bags, wipe down the bottom once a week with a paper towel that's been lightly sprayed with an all-purpose sanitizing spray. (Test an area first to make sure your bag is color-safe.) Hang your bag up whenever possible (why does it always seem that the bathroom stall I pick is missing its hook?) and try using a purse hook to keep your bag off the floor in restaurants (you can find chic ones at luxelink.com).

Give that cell phone or PDA a once-weekly wipe with an all-purpose cleanser or hand sanitizer. They can pick up a nasty mix of lipstick, saliva, and food particles.

Keep some hand sanitizer in your purse for on-the-go de-germing after handling money, riding the subway, taking your kids to the playground, shaking hands with that clammy chick in marketing, or handling food. EO (eoproducts.com) makes a great line of hand-sanitizing gels, sprays, and wipes that don't dry out your skin like those from a lot of other brands.

Germ-Free Shopping

See that cart that you're about to grab? Hundreds of people have touched the handle today already.[24] Some kid probably had his poopy tushy right where you're about to place your raw spinach. Go ahead and clean off the handle with the antibacterial wipes that most stores now supply. You can even bring your own dishwasher-safe handle cover (like Healthy Handle) to the store. It may sound over-the-top, but if you have a little one, you might want to bring one of the new handy cart covers that allow you to create your own safe little environment for picking up the groceries. Design your own with really great fabric (no neon dancing clowns here) at www.just-peachybaby.com.

Belly Tip

Bag lady. Instead of lugging your purse all over your house with you—and ostensibly spreading around any germs it might be harboring—create a landing spot (I use a wall hook) for it by your front door. That way you won't be tempted to sling it onto your bedspread or drop it on your kitchen counter. Bonus— you'll never have to ask where the hell your purse is.

Now that the cart itself is clean as a whistle, let's keep the food in good shape. Load up all your produce and nonperishables first (cereal, canned beans, pasta sauce, etc.), and then hit the dairy and meat aisles. You want those items to stay cold for as long as possible. Grab a plastic bag to cover packages of meat and poultry, which will help prevent those icky juices from seeping out onto your fresh berries. Make the frozen aisle your last stop before checkout.

If you live far from the store or plan to make several stops on the way home, it's a good idea to keep an insulated bag or cooler in the car. Transfer meats, milk, yogurt, eggs, and other chilled items into the cooler before driving home. Once you're home, get those frozen and perishable items put away first.

It seems like a whole lot to remember to stay safe, but it's really just common sense. Get some soap, hand sanitizer, and antibacterial wipes, and you'll be all set. Remember, just washing your hands with regular soap is the number one thing you can do to ditch germs.

Chapter Fifteen

Belly in the Kitchen

It's getting a bit tough to see your feet these days, and you may have noticed that you're not as nimble as you used to be. The place where that can really come into play is the kitchen. Being pregnant doesn't make cooking more difficult or more dangerous; it just means you'll need to do a few things differently.

Be Sweet to Your Feet

Make yourself comfortable. The extra weight and fluid you're carrying means that your ankles may be swollen at the end of the day (cankle alert!), so try to put your feet up for at least ten minutes when you get home.

Make sure to change into comfortable shoes before cooking dinner, but don't go for something totally flat, like flip-flops. Your shoes should be non-skid and include an arch support, says Dr. Marlene Reid, a podiatric surgeon in Westmont, Illinois.[1]

What about those cool cooking clogs that all the chefs wear? As long as they have a back, they're fine. Open-backed shoes of any kind offer less stability. Here's a good test for stability from Dr. Reid: Hold the shoe in both hands and bend it front to back. It should bend at the ball of the foot, not at the arch. Next, twist the shoe laterally in two different directions. It shouldn't give.[2] So all those cutesy ballet flats that are so popular aren't really the best thing for your feet right now.

Choose shoes made of natural materials, like leather, suede, and fabric, because they move with you and breathe better. Thicker straps are better than skinny ones, which can cut into your skin when you're swollen. If you're having a lot of heel or arch pain, see a podiatrist about getting custom orthotics for your shoes.[3]

Another word on shoes: Since your feet can grow up to a size larger during pregnancy—and stay that way—now is *not* the time to invest in Jimmy Choos or an amazing pair of boots. I'd hate to see them not fit you at the bris or christening.

Take a Load Off

Give those puffy legs and feet a break and try sitting for certain tasks, such as chopping and peeling. When you need to pick things up, make sure to bend from your knees instead of your back (really good advice for when you're not preggers, too). Since your belly will be increasingly in the way and prone to getting dripped on and splattered, treat yourself to a fun new apron. Marimekko, Anthropologie, and Kitch n' Glam make fabulous ones that will grow with you. It might sound silly, but wearing something fun might help inspire you to keep cooking (or at least whipping up healthy smoothies) during those last few weeks of pregnancy.

Just like you can get overheated during exercise, cooking can make your temperature rise. Open a window or keep a fan blowing to help keep the air circulating. If you feel overheated or light-headed, sit down and drink some water. Keep a tall glass of water handy while you're cooking to stay hydrated.

Your center of gravity has changed, and your back can feel like you've been doing hours of intense weeding.[4] Don't pull that heavy roast out of the oven by yourself; ask someone else to do it. Instead of climbing up on the counter to reach that can of beans or dust the top of the fridge, pass the buck.

Basic Kitchen Training

If it were up to me everyone would take a course on basic knife skills. When you don't know what you're supposed to do with one, a knife—especially a 6- or 7-inch chef's knife—can seem really scary. But when you know how to hold one and use it properly, a knife is your most useful kitchen tool.

Here's how to hold a knife: Look at your knife. There's a seam where the handle meets the blade. Place your thumb near the seam on one side of the knife and your index finger on the opposite side, so you're pinching the blade between those two fingers. Your other three fingers should be curled up and wrapped around the knife's handle. If you've never held a knife this way before, it will feel odd, but it's the safest and most effective way to hold a knife. It gives you a ton more control as you slice through food.

Now that you know how to hold a knife, here are some tips for using it:

- **Make sure it's sharp**. Dullness is usually what causes you to slip up and cut yourself. You can sharpen your knives with a sharpening steel or stone. If you don't want to do it yourself, find a service to do it for you. If your knives are crappy and you've had them since college, it's probably time for an upgrade anyway.

- **Get a grip**. Some women find that they just don't like the heft of a traditional steel blade. If you're in that camp, you might want to try a ceramic knife, such as the ones made by Kyocera. I love them. They're super-sharp, light, and feel really good in my tiny hand. The only downsides are that they can't be sharpened like steel blades, and if you drop them, they're liable to chip.

- **Be square**. Instead of cutting through round things that like to roll, like carrots and squash, square them off first by cutting off the sides or ends. Then you'll have a nice, stable base. I'm not talking about turning a round vegetable into a square one—just cut off a little on one side so that the flat side can rest on your cutting board safely while you slice through the vegetable.

- **Store safely**. Keep knives in a knife block or on a magnetic strip, which has the added bonus of looking amazingly cool on your wall. Never store your knives (unless they're small paring knives) in a drawer. They'll get dull, and you'll risk nicking yourself each time you reach for one. However you store them, make sure they're out of the reach of little ones.

- **Hand wash**. Putting good knives in the dishwasher is a no-no. They can become dull and the tips can bend. Many knives have wooden handles that can loosen over time, which again makes them less safe to use. At about $100 a pop for a good knife, you'll want yours to last a long time. A quick scrub under hot, soapy water is all you need to clean your good knives. Butter knives and small knives with plastic handles will hold up in the dishwasher just fine.

Chapter Sixteen

Momma Munchies

Feel like you just had breakfast and yet you're already hungry? That's pretty much how it goes once you finally get past morning sickness. I remember eating a small snack before starting my forty-five-minute commute to work and then being ravenous by the time I got to the office. If you're expecting multiples, your hunger is kicked into even higher gear. To make sure you're not hitting up vending machines or spending half your life in the kitchen, get savvy about snacking. You want things that can be put together quickly, keep you satisfied, *and* supply all those nutrients you and your baby bump need. Since they're supposed to be snacks, they should be small enough to not ruin your next meal.

Momma Munchies—Great Anytime Snacks[1]

Snack	Calories
½ whole-wheat bagel or 4 whole-grain crackers (like Kashi TLC) + 1 tablespoon peanut or almond butter	230
1 cup jicama sticks + 2 tablespoons guacamole	103
¼ cup nuts + ¼ cup dried fruit	306

1 medium organic apple +
1-ounce slice of aged cheddar cheese   173

1 8-ounce glass of organic reduced-fat
chocolate milk   195

1 organic cheese stick + 1 small orange   120
(the cheese stick solo is 80 calories)

6 ounces organic vanilla yogurt +
1 tablespoon wheat germ + ½ cup berries   154

½ avocado (mashed) + 1 piece rye crisp bread,
like Wasa   197

2 Fig Newtons (preferably whole-grain) +
1 teaspoon almond butter   149

1 whole-grain tortilla + ½ cup halved cherry
tomatoes + 2 tablespoons hummus   205

4 ounces (snack size) low-fat (1%) organic
cottage cheese + ½ cup cubed cantaloupe +
2 tablespoons granola   152

½ English muffin + 1 tablespoon
golden raisins + ½ cup sliced apples +
1 tablespoon peanut butter   285

Make-your-own trail mix: 1 tablespoon
pumpkin seeds + 1 tablespoon dried cherries +
1 tablespoon dried cranberries +
1 tablespoon almonds   166

1 ounce walnuts (14 halves)   185

1 small, 4-inch whole-wheat pita +
1 hard-boiled DHA-fortified egg, chopped   152

1 cup baby carrots + ¼ cup All-Purpose
Veggie Dip (page 232)   102

Special Foods for Moms-to-Be

I always go for homemade over processed foods, but in our crazy, hectic world, you sometimes need a backup plan. Now, there are some tasty and healthy snacks that are formulated for a mom-to-be's needs. They're a bit pricey ($2.40 a bar and up), but if you're on the go and want to avoid the fast-food and fatty-muffin traps, they can be a lifesaver. Here are ones I've taste-tested and think are worth the money:

Belly Bar (find its products at Whole Foods, Target, and many other stores) makes bars, shakes, and chews. The bars taste pretty good and have 200 percent of the folic acid you need each day. Plus, they're low in saturated fat, are trans fat-free, and have a vegetarian source of DHA (see page 74), a form of omega-3 that has been shown to play a role in a baby's brain development. Belly Bar's awesome little chews are only 20 calories each and come in citrus (they taste like Starburst!) and chocolate flavors.

Oh Mama! Bars and Ginger Ale Elixir. Unless it's the middle of summer, these bars should be fine in the glove compartment of your car for a week or so. DHAs are heat sensitive, so make sure to keep an eye on the sell-by date. The ginger ale is made with real ginger and has 400 mcg of folic acid, plus vitamin B6.

> **Belly Tip**
>
> **Act like your grandmother.** Start hoarding snacks in your purse. (Why else are you carrying around that enormous bag?) Stock up at your desk and in your car, while you're at it. Of course, these will have to be non-perishable snacks, such as crackers, pretzels, and dried fruit. To help you stick to the portion size, measure out servings of nuts, baby carrots, graham crackers, etc., on Sunday, so they're ready to go for the rest of the week. Use 1-ounce zip-lock bags or small plastic containers. They'll be easier to add to your purse or lunch bag, and you won't risk eating your way through a whole bag of nuts.

Avoiding Drive-Thru Disasters

When that hunger starts hitting you like a ton of bricks around month four (or even during your first trimester to fight morning sickness), you'll have moments where you're suddenly drawn to naughty, greasy foods, just like you were drawn to that rebellious new boy back in ninth grade. Like high school, there will most certainly be things you'll regret. You know that fast food isn't your best option, but is any of it okay, or even nutritious? It's never going to be your healthiest option, simply because of all the preservatives and sodium added to the food to make it taste good, but it can be a fairly healthy pick when other options are limited. And one really good thing about fast-food spots is that they almost always offer cartons of plain and chocolate milk, which can be tough to find at more upscale places.

Plus, fast-food chains are becoming better about offering up in-store nutrition info (New York City now requires that all fast-food places include nutrition info front and center, and other cities are following suit), and you can pretty much always find the info online. These days, it's easy to look up your favorite

Belly Tip

Nighttime nibbles. Toward the end of your pregnancy, when your belly and breasts are heaving and you feel like you're about to pop, sleep can become elusive. Even though you're dog-tired, it's tough to find a comfortable position—or at least a position that stays comfortable. Plus, your need to pee more frequently just keeps getting worse, so even when you do drift off for a few sweet minutes, your bladder ends up waking you. And even though he hasn't officially arrived, Baby is definitely making his presence known with little prize-fighter jabs inside your belly.

While there's not a whole lot you can do other than try to make yourself comfy with special pillows and maybe a warm bath or shower before bed, there are certain snacks that might send you off to Dreamland a bit more quickly. The combination of the amino acid tryptophan and carbohydrates can help make you drowsy.[2] Some combinations include home-cooked roasted turkey on a slice of whole-grain bread, a glass of milk and a cookie, cheese and crackers, and hummus on a pita. If you've been having trouble sleeping, a small snack like this about thirty to forty minutes before bed may be just the ticket.

items before you go to see how they compare. I've rounded up the smartest picks for your belly below.

Arby's

Meat cravings might have you pulling up to this joint. If you choose right, you can maximize protein and iron and minimize fat and sodium in your meal.

Regular Roast Beef Sandwich on a Sesame Bun with Horsey Sauce (skip the sauce and you'll cut out 173 mg sodium):

382 calories, 18 g fat (7 g saturated, 0.5 g trans), 49 mg cholesterol, 1,126 mg sodium, 20 g protein

Martha's Vineyard Salad

276 calories, 8 g fat (4 saturated, 0 trans fat), 72 mg cholesterol, 452 mg sodium, 26 g protein

McDonald's

It's known for helping fatten up the nation's waistline, and there's one in pretty much every small town and urban area in the country. When it's the best bet around, here's what to get.

Premium Asian Salad with Grilled Chicken (get it without the orange glaze and you'll save on sodium and sugar):

300 calories, 10 g fat (1 g saturated), 65 mg cholesterol, 890 mg sodium, 5 g fiber, 32 g protein, 140 mg calcium, 2.5 mg iron

Egg McMuffin (order it without the Canadian-style bacon and the liquid margarine and you'll save on sodium and fat):

300 calories, 12 g fat (5 g saturated), 260 mg cholesterol, 820 mg sodium, 18 g protein, 160 mg calcium, 2 mg iron

Fruit 'n' Yogurt Parfait with Granola

160 calories, 2 g fat (1 g saturated), 5 mg cholesterol, 85 mg cholesterol, 4 g protein, 130 mg calcium

Wendy's

This chain boasts that its burgers are always fresh, not frozen. And who doesn't love a Frosty? There are some decent picks here, but you need to know what to go for.

Broccoli and Cheese Baked Potato

320 calories, 2 g fat (1.5 g saturated, 0 g trans), 5 mg cholesterol, 450 mg sodium, 8 g fiber, 10 g protein, 10 percent daily calcium

Chicken Caesar Salad (skip the croutons and only use one packet of Caesar dressing; if you can be really good, skip the dressing altogether)

305 calories, 19 g fat (4.75 g saturated), 87.5 mg cholesterol, 855 mg sodium, 3 g fiber, 25 g protein, 20 percent daily calcium

Grilled Chicken Go Wrap

260 calories, 11 g fat (3.5 g saturated), 45 mg cholesterol, 760 mg cholesterol, 17 g protein

Burger King

Again, no one is saying that BK is a health-food restaurant. Far from it, but if you find yourself there at some point, a few items do pass muster:

Whopper Junior without mayo (BK does offer veggie burgers, but they're actually higher in calories and sodium, which is a bummer)

290 calories, 12 g fat (4.5 saturated, 0.5 trans), 35 mg cholesterol, 500 mg sodium, 2 g fiber, 16 g protein, 3.6 mg iron

Tendergrill Garden Salad with Ken's Light Italian dressing, no croutons (use less dressing or take off some of the cheese to reduce the sodium and fat)

360 calories, 20 g fat (5 g saturated, 0 g trans), 80 mg cholesterol, 1,160 mg sodium, 5 g fiber, 33 g protein, 2.7 mg iron

Beyond the Drive-Thru

These days there are a lot of places that offer quick options but aren't considered part of the fast-food landscape. You'll see more ethnic-inspired options here, and lots and lots of drinks.

Au Bon Pain

This is a great airport choice. Au Bon Pain has a fun "Portions" menu that lets you indulge in small servings of tasty items, such as BBQ chicken, cheddar cheese, fruit, and crackers. All of the Portions are around 200 calories, so they're a perfect fix for late afternoon hunger. The restaurants also have flavorful soups that aren't loaded with sodium (the Old Fashioned Tomato Rice soup has 340 mg), and healthy breakfast items like oatmeal and yogurt with fruit.

Panera

Tasty salads and "You Pick Two" options that allow you to get half a sandwich and a cup of soup or a salad are great healthy choices. Plus, this spot is super kid-friendly, so if you already have a little one, it's a nice place to go and relax for a millisecond. Panera also offers breakfast options, like a grilled egg and cheese sandwich with all-natural eggs and Vermont cheddar. I'm a fan because Panera has lots of nice whole-grain bread options.

Chipotle

This McDonald's-owned chain has done an amazing job of sourcing natural, hormone-free meats, organic beans, and hormone-free sour cream. The burritos are really tasty, but downing an entire one in a sitting is a recipe for heartburn. Even though you get to choose what goes into your burrito, it's almost always going to add up to 800 calories or more. Eat half and take the rest home for dinner.

Trade in that 330-calorie burrito wrap for a burrito bowl and you're automatically cutting calories. Load up on the fajita veggies, lean meats, and beans, and choose either the sour cream *or* cheese on top. The tacos are another great option because they're made from whole-grain corn. In addition, Chipotle is now sourcing some of its produce locally, so the romaine lettuce in your burrito will be fresher than if it came from halfway across the country.

Dunkin' Donuts

This national chain was once only known for its sugar-bomb donuts and cheap coffee, but it's gotten savvy and now offers a DDSmart menu. Its toasted Egg and Cheese on English Muffin, with 310 calories and 13 g fat (5 g saturated), is a better bet than getting a sandwich on a bagel or croissant, but it does have a substantial 1,300 mg sodium, so go easy on the salt the rest of the day. Even lighter is the Egg-White Veggie Flatbread sandwich, with 290 calories, 9 g fat (4 g saturated), and a more reasonable 680 mg sodium. By the way, both sandwiches have fewer calories than any of Dunkin's muffins.

Starbucks

Yes, Starbucks still has the typical coffeehouse options, such as muffins, bagels, and scones, but it recently beefed up its healthy options. Starbucks now serves oatmeal for breakfast and baked goods that are low in fat and rich in fiber. I'm a big fan of the Baked Berry Stella (280 calories, 9 g fat, 6 g fiber) and the cheese, fruit, and protein plate. And while they are pretty high in sodium, the English muffin-based breakfast sandwiches can be a good choice. Most locations also sell small bags of roasted almonds, which I almost always carry in my purse.

Plus, with Starbucks' Vivanno Nourishing Blends smoothie options, you can start your day with something other than decaf coffee or tea. Each 250-calorie Vivanno smoothie boasts a whole banana, plus whey protein and added fiber, in each serving.

Jamba Juice

Speaking of smoothies, they're a fabulous thing when you're pregnant because you can pack a lot of nutrients into one glass and sneak in goodies like calcium. It's easy to make a really healthy smoothie at home, like the ones that start on page 249. There are lots of places to find them on the go to, but you really have to watch out for the portion size. Jamba Juice's smallest size is 12 ounces and goes up to a whopping 30 ounces. No one needs this much smoothie—or the 600 calories that can come with it—ever!

Stick with the smallest size, and go with the fewest fancy options. At the same time, you probably shouldn't choose straight-up, fresh-squeezed juices, because they're unpasteurized, which means that the juice could carry bacteria. It's not really a huge deal when you're not pregnant, but your immune system isn't quite up to snuff now. And remember to steer clear of their energy boosts that include the stimulants guarana, ginseng, and green tea. Jamba Juice also offers dairy, gluten-free, and vegan options, which is nice.

If you're at Smoothie King, Robeks, or a neighborhood juice joint, stick to the same advice.

Belly Up to the Bar

For the true on-the-go mini-meal, hardly anything beats the convenience of an energy bar or granola bar, but many fall short on taste and nutrition. Their two biggest issues are saturated fat and sugar. Go for ones that don't have yogurt or chocolate coatings—that's what runs up the saturated fat tally (stick to bars with 3 g or less and no trans fat). A good bar should have 7 to 10 g protein and a few grams of fiber. Of course, plenty of choices abound. Here are the top picks:

Clif

One of the first bars to go the more natural route, these chunky, satisfying, 70-percent-organic bars don't have a laundry list of ingredients and taste more like a homemade cookie than many overly processed options. Clif bars usually hover around the 250-calorie mark with 10 g protein from soy, 20 g sugar, and a decent amount of folic acid. Fat ranges from 3 to 6 g, with as much as 2 g of saturated fat. They're a bit more than what you'd need for a snack, but if you need to make it from 3 p.m. until dinner and can't find yogurt and a piece of fruit, it's your next-best bet.

Larabar

While not a heavyweight in the protein department, this bar is fabulous because it's barely processed (just nuts, dried fruit, spices, and sometimes chocolate). The Ginger Snap flavor might even help calm a queasy stomach. Most flavors are about 220 calories, 5 g fiber, 5 g protein, 1 g saturated fat, and zero trans fat. Bonus: Larabars are completely gluten-free.

Luna and Luna Sunrise

Made especially for women, they're packed with folic acid and calcium. Plus, they're only 180 calories. And Luna Sunrise bars also contain vitamin D.

YouBars

Haven't found one you like yet? Make your own! I'm not talking about spending hours in the kitchen. Just go to www.youbars.com and custom blend a bar that suits your picky tastes. You start with a base of various nut butters (if you have tree nut, peanut, or soy allergies, these bars are not for you), then add extra goodies like dried fruits, protein powder, nuts, seeds, and natural sweeteners, such as honey and molasses. Be sure to leave out the optional vitamin infusions, as they may be overload when coupled with your prenatal vitamin. As you build your bars, you can see how the nutritional information stacks up.

The price tag might seem a little hefty ($40 for a case), but you're getting exactly what you want in a bar. Think of it as a much less pricey alternative to custom couture. If you don't like the bar you concocted, they'll let you order another box at no charge.

Chapter Seventeen

Recipes to Feed the Belly

Finally, after all this talk, we're getting to the good stuff! I've organized the *Feed the Belly* recipes by craving: Sweet, Meaty, Salty/Savory, Spicy, and Thirst-Quenching. Craving something salty? Turn to the Salty/Savory section on page 208—maybe my Pesto Pizza will hit the spot.

Each recipe includes either a **Baby Bonus**—an extra nutrient that helps Baby develop—or a **Momma Must-Have**—a goodie that keeps you feeling healthy, happy, and strong. Many have both. You can also look up recipes based on the nutrients they contain. Just found out you're anemic? Go to the Baby Bonus index on page 152 to find recipes rich in folate, protein, calcium, iron, and so on.

I've designed most of the recipes to serve four. I figure that if you're going to go to the trouble to cook, you'll probably want leftovers. If not, the recipes can easily be halved. I call for convenience ingredients, such as canned beans and bagged cabbage, where I think it makes sense, and I offer tips for making the recipes faster. Here's the thing—making food at home is always going to be the healthiest (and cheapest) way to go, because you know exactly what's going into each dish and can control the amount of sodium, fat, and sugar, and use organic and natural ingredients. But hey, sometimes the thought of handling meat or pulling out pots and pans seems like as much fun as caulking the tub. That's fine too. I'm hoping these recipes can also inspire you to make healthier decisions when you're dining out.

Where I think it makes a difference, I've called for organic ingredients (usually dairy and meat, and often produce). If you can't find organic or would rather not use it, that's fine. Macaroni and cheese with conventional cheese instead of organic cheese will work just as well.

If you're working full time or you already have little ones in the house, it can be incredibly tough to whip up dinner each night. Lack of time and sheer exhaustion can derail even the most Martha types. Try to plan your meals ahead of time and shop and cook on Sundays. That way, you'll know you can at least eat home-cooked meals through Tuesday. And if you're super-organized, you can make double batches of things you really like and freeze them.

Tips on Freezing Foods

Oxygen is the enemy of food. Keep it out with freezer bags or vacuum-sealing systems like Foodsaver. I really like the Handi-Vac from Reynolds because it doesn't take up counter space and is easy to use.

Use **a permanent marker to list the date the food was cooked and the contents** of the package. Once it's two to three months old, throw it out. This works especially well when you've had a craving for something—say, chili—made a ton of it, and then just couldn't stand the thought of it. Who knows? Maybe in two weeks, you'll be lusting for it again. For a complete list of refrigerator and freezer storage times, go to http://www.cfsan.fda.gov/~pregnant/refrfrez.pdf.

Keep ice cream and frozen yogurt fresher by **putting a piece of plastic wrap over the top of the ice cream** before placing the lid back on. It'll help keep the air out, which is the culprit behind that horrible freezer-burn taste. Of course, if you go through ice cream like my husband and I do, there's not much time for the flavor to go bad.

Okay, I think you're armed with more than enough information. Now go forth and cook! Your belly will thank you for it.

Sweet

"The bottom line for me was cravings for a lot of sweet things, and I rarely eat sweets. I even wanted those really fatty, sugary, as-big-as-your-head muffins from time to time."—**Andrea**

Chocolatey

Better Than Elvis Milkshake (omega-3s, folic acid, calcium)

Chunky Monkey Muffins (protein, bran for extra fiber, omega-3 from flax seeds)

Extra-Chocolatey Cupcakes (calcium, antioxidants)

Oh! Susannah Chocolate Maltshake (calcium, vitamin A)

Citrusy

Pucker Up Mini Lemon Tartlets (only 80 calories!)

Meyer Lemon Granita (great cure for nausea and very low cal)

Citrus-Spiked Rice Pudding (calcium, fiber)

Creamy

Carrot Cake Dream Bars (beta-carotene, fiber)

Oatmeal Brulée (fiber, calcium)

Mornin' Sunshine Parfait (protein, calcium)

Sweet Baby Bread Pudding (rich in calcium and lower in fat than most bread puddings, and it just *rocks!*)

Walnut-Maple Syrup Sauce with Vanilla Ice Cream (decadent treat with healthy omega-3s)

Fruity

Deconstructed Apple Pie (high fiber, antioxidant-rich)

Fresh Fruit with Creamy Yo-Co Dip (vitamin C, omega-3 from flax seeds)

Fruity Booty Salad (potassium, fiber)

Peach and Blackberry Crumble (fiber, beta-carotene)

Salty/Sweet

Baby on Board Banana Bread (potassium, calcium, fiber)

Hippie-Chick Granola (fiber, plus heart-healthy pumpkin seeds, oats, almonds, and other goodies)

Morning, Noon, and Night Nut Clusters (nutty satisfaction for just 60 calories)

Oh, Baby! Breakfast Cookies (antioxidants and indulgence in an absolutely guilt-free treat)

Meaty

"During the first trimester, even before I knew I was pregnant, I was crazed for meat. RED MEAT. I'm not generally a big meat eater at all, and I very rarely eat red meat. But when I was pregnant, I found myself stopping off for cheeseburgers during the drive home from work, and then cooking steaks for dinner. My body went completely cave girl on me."—**Renée**

Red Meat, Poultry, Pork

Chicken Pot Pie (protein, iron)

Koto Kapama (Cinnamon-Stewed Chicken) (protein, iron, zinc)

Lemony Chicken with Capers (superfast!)

Mini Meatballs with Kale and Orecchiette (protein, iron, beta-carotene, folate)

Momma's Meatloaf (protein, iron, calcium; guilt-free comfort food)

Pork Chops with Asparagus and Morels (protein, choline)

Tuscan Turkey Burgers (protein, iron, calcium, fiber)

Seafood

Baked Mediterranean Tilapia (protein, omega-3, less than 300 calories)

Ginger-Glazed Salmon (omega-3; super-fast!)

Shrimp with Peas and Pesto (folate, omega-3, calcium)

Vegetarian

Everything but the Kitchen Sink Frittata (protein, choline, folate, beta-carotene)

Ginger Egg Fried Rice (fiber; super-fast!)

Salty/Savory

"With Kate, my second born, I could not get enough protein, veggies, and salty ethnic food. And I just couldn't eat enough cheese."—**Heidi**

Salads

Confetti Rice Salad (calcium, fiber)

Roasted Beet, Pistachio, and Goat Cheese Salad with Basil Vinaigrette (folate, fiber, calcium)

Spinach and Pear Salad with Pomegranate Dressing (antioxidants, omega-3, beta-carotene, potassium)

Mediterranean Barley Salad (iron, zinc, fiber)

The Wedge (calcium; less than 100 calories!)

Warm Fig Salad with Pecans (fiber, potassium)

Mustardy Green Bean and Cherry Tomato Salad (folate, beta-carotene)

Soups

Miso Pretty Soup (zinc for immunity, calcium)

Roasted Fall Vegetable Soup (beta-carotene, vitamin C, fiber)

Sweetie-Pie Sweet Potato Soup (beta-carotene, potassium)

Pastas

Brocco Mac and Cheese (calcium, fiber; major comfort food!)

Farfalle with Edamame and Pecorino (protein, fiber, folate, calcium)

Vegetable Sides

Roasted Spring Asparagus (folate, vitamin D)

Smashed Edamame and Potatoes with Miso (potassium, fiber)

Mean Greens and Beans (calcium, beta-carotene, fiber, iron)

Grilled Vegetables in the Style of Santa Margherita (vitamin C, fiber)

Other Tasty Things

All-Purpose Veggie Dip (calcium)

Pesto Pizza Pie (calcium, fiber)

Matzah Brei (protein, vitamin B_{12})

Spicy

"When I was pregnant with Bennett, it was the spicier, the better for me. But that was only after my first trimester, when all I could eat was plain noodles and baked potatoes."—**Brandi**

Main Dishes

Alisa's Taco Salad with Yogurty Salsa (protein, iron, zinc, fiber)

Huevos Rancheros Wrap (protein, choline, iron)

Not-Too-Spicy Thai Chicken Curry (protein, potassium, iron, fiber)

Pregnancy Pad Thai (calcium, folate, iron)

Soups and Veggies

Peasant-Style Gazpacho (vitamin C, lycopene)

Rainy Day Chili (protein, iron, fiber)

Sesame-Ginger Green Beans (fiber)

Thirst-Quenching

"I was so thirsty when I was pregnant, which was frustrating because there weren't a lot of decaf drink options. I really craved lemonade and anything refreshing."
—**Brooke**

Dairy

Nana–Berry Smoothie (potassium, protein, calcium)

Renée's Orange Creamsicle (vitamin C, calcium)

Non-Dairy

Gingery Watermelon Liquado (lycopene)

Le Royale (refreshing mocktail)

Love That Bump Lemonade (great morning sickness antidote)

Mango-Pineapple Crush (vitamin C)

Papaya-Blue Lagoon (folate, antioxidants, vitamin C)

SWEET

CHOCOLATEY

Better Than Elvis Milkshake

This yummy milkshake is packed with baby-building nutrients. If you like it thicker, add 4 ounces of plain low-fat yogurt. It's nutrient-rich, but also calorie-packed and can be used as a meal when you don't have time to sit down for a proper one. Split it if you only need a snack. You can make twice the amount and store in the fridge in an airtight container (sports bottles work well) for a day. Just make sure to shake it up again before drinking.

Prep time: 5 minutes

Makes 1 serving (about 10 ounces)

Baby Bonus: Shake it, baby, because this one is loaded with bennies! It has a boatload of omega-3 fats from the soy milk and wheat germ, plus more than 30 percent of your daily calcium needs. It's also got more than 20 percent of your folic acid requirement, and a significant amount of other B vitamins.

Momma Must-Have: It's yummy, chocolatey, and very decadent. Need I say more?

8 ounces omega-3-enhanced soy milk

1 teaspoon toasted wheat germ

2 tablespoons low-sugar Nesquik

½ of a medium banana

2 tablespoons natural peanut butter

1. Place all ingredients into a blender. Blend on high until smooth.

2. Serve in a tall glass. If you like it really cold, add a few ice cubes.

Calories 404; Fat 21 g (Sat 2.5 g, Mono 9 g, Poly 9 g, Omega-3 302 mg); Cholesterol
0 mg; Protein 7 g; Carbohydrate 9 g; Sugars 27 g; Fiber 5 g; Iron 2 mg; Sodium
241 mg; Calcium 367 mg; Folate 135 mcg

Chunky Monkey Muffins

My goal for this recipe was to create a chocolatey banana muffin. This definitely fits the bill, and it's also great for those
times when things aren't moving so well...if you know what I
mean. Each muffin has 3 grams of fiber, so eat it with a full
glass of water and grab some reading material. If you like a tasty
little surprise in your baked goods, add a dollop of peanut buttery
goodness inside.

Prep: 10 minutes

Cook: 20 minutes

Makes 15 muffins

Baby Bonus: 5 grams of protein means this muffin has way more
than empty calories—plus, it's got a bit of vegetarian omega-3
from the flax seeds.

Momma Must-Have: 3 grams of fiber.

1¼ cups organic whole-wheat flour

½ cup all-purpose flour

¾ cup packed brown sugar

2 tablespoons ground flax seed

1 tablespoon, plus 1 teaspoon, dark cocoa powder
(such as Hershey's Special Dark)

2 teaspoons baking soda

¼ teaspoon salt

⅔ cup semisweet chocolate chips

6 ounces low-fat organic vanilla yogurt

2 medium overripe bananas, mashed

1 egg (preferably omega-3-enhanced)

1 teaspoon vanilla extract

2 tablespoons vegetable oil

¼ cup soy or organic 1% milk

⅓ cup natural smooth peanut butter (optional)

1 tablespoon (or more) wheat germ

1. Preheat oven to 350°F. Line a 12-cup muffin tin with paper liners. Coat liners with cooking spray and set aside.

2. Measure out the flours, leveling with a knife, into a large mixing bowl along with the brown sugar, flax seed, 1 tablespoon cocoa powder, baking soda, salt, and chocolate chips. Whisk together until combined.

3. Combine the yogurt, bananas, egg, vanilla extract, oil, and soy milk in a separate bowl until thoroughly mixed (it's okay if there are a few chunks of banana left).

4. Fold the banana mixture into the dry mixture just until combined. If using peanut butter, fill the prepared muffin cups ½ full with batter and then spoon 1 teaspoon peanut butter on top. Fill the cups with more batter until ¾ full (if not using peanut butter, simply fill the cups ¾ full with batter). Sprinkle tops with wheat germ and put in the oven for 20 minutes or until the tops of the muffins look dry and spring back when touched in the center. Allow to cool on the stovetop.

5. Bake the remaining muffin mixture while you're snacking on a warm one, and go find a good magazine.

Calories 240; Fat 9 g (Sat 3 g, Mono 0.5 g, Poly 2 g); Cholesterol 15 mg; Protein 5 g; Carbohydrate 36 g; Sugars 15 g; Fiber 3 g; Iron 1 mg; Sodium 246 mg; Calcium 32 mg

Extra Chocolatey Cupcakes

Gale Gand is truly a superwoman. She's the executive pastry chef and a partner at Tru, Osteria di Tramonto, Gale's Coffee Bar, Tramonto's Steak & Seafood, and RT Lounge, all Chicago-area restaurants; host of the Food Network show *Sweet Dreams*, a cookbook author, and mom of three. When Gale was pregnant with her twin girls, Ella and Ruby, she got her chocolate fix with these cupcakes. They are truly a chocolatey indulgence. The boiling water activates the baking soda and helps keep the cupcakes moist.

Prep: 5 minutes

Cook: 25 minutes

Makes 12 servings

Momma Must-Have: This is moist, rich, and chocolatey heaven! Instead of digging into a slice of double-chocolate cake and racking up around 900 calories, soothe your chocolate demons for less than 300 calories with this decadent-tasting cupcake.

1 cup organic white sugar

1 cup organic brown sugar

1¼ cups all-purpose flour

½ cup whole-wheat flour

¾ cup unsweetened cocoa powder

1 ½ teaspoons baking powder

1 ½ teaspoons baking soda

1 teaspoon salt

2 eggs

1 cup whole milk

½ cup vegetable oil

1 teaspoon pure vanilla extract

1 teaspoon almond extract

1 cup boiling water

Confectioners' sugar, for dusting

1. Preheat the oven to 375°F. Line a 12-count muffin tin with paper muffin cups.

2. Combine the sugars, flours, cocoa powder, baking powder, baking soda, and salt together in a stand mixer fitted with a whisk attachment on medium speed (you can use a hand mixer instead).

3. Add the eggs and milk, and mix till well combined. Drizzle in the oil and the vanilla and almond extracts and mix again. With the mixer running at low speed, add the boiling water and mix just until smooth. The batter will be thin.

4. Fill the lined muffin cups about ⅔ full. Bake until cupcakes rise and are firm to the touch, about 25 to 30 minutes. Let cool in the pans. Dust with confectioners' sugar, if desired.

Calories 287; Fat 12 g (Sat 2.5 g, Mono 2.5 g, Poly 6 g); Cholesterol 39 mg; Protein 5 g; Carbohydrate 13 g; Sugars 31 g; Fiber 3 g; Iron 2 mg; Sodium 431 mg; Calcium 79 mg; Folate 21 mcg

Oh! Susannah Chocolate Maltshake

When my friend Susannah was pregnant with her daughter, Thalia, she went on a quest for chocolate malteds. Not finding any in the Birmingham, Alabama, area, she took matters into her own hands. If you're curious, malted milk powder is made from evaporated versions of malted barley, wheat flour, and whole milk powder. In case you're craving that chocolatey—and decidedly malty—flavor, give this recipe a spin. At the very least, it's bound to make you feel like a little girl again. Like Susannah, you may just want to put your hair in pigtails before you take a sip.

Prep: 5 minutes

Makes 2 8-ounce shakes (but you might want it all for yourself)

Baby Bonus: Nearly 30 percent of calcium and 50 percent of vitamin A daily requirements.

Momma Must-Have: It's got a ton of potassium to help relieve middle-of-the-night leg cramps. It's great for those times when you're trying to pack in more calcium, but just can't stomach another glass of milk.

1 cup low-fat double-churned vanilla ice cream

1 tablespoon malted milk powder (such as Carnation)

1 tablespoon dark chocolate syrup (try to find one fortified with extra calcium)

1 cup 1% organic or soy milk

1. Place all ingredients in a blender, and blend until smooth. Pour into a tall glass, with ice if you like, and serve with a fun straw.

Calories 240; Fat 9 g (Sat 3 g, Mono 0.5 g, Poly 2 g); Cholesterol 15 mg; Protein 5 g; Carbohydrate 36 g; Sugars 15 g; Fiber 3 g; Iron 1 mg; Sodium 246 mg; Calcium 32 mg

CITRUSY

Pucker Up Mini Lemon Tartlets

One of my favorite flavor combos is lemon and coconut. In fact, my wedding cake was lemon and coconut, and boy, was it rich. These super-light, petite bites give you the same hit of tangy-sweet but with a fraction of the sugar and calories. They're only 80 calories for two!

Prep: 7 minutes

Cook: 7 minutes

Makes 24 tartlets (2 per serving)

Momma Must-Have: Tame your citrus craving for just 80 calories a serving!

6 tablespoons fat-free sweetened condensed milk

2 egg yolks

1½ teaspoons grated lemon zest (about 1 lemon)

2 tablespoons fresh lemon juice

24 mini pastry shells
(such as Clearbrook Farms
Mini Sweet Tart Shells)

¼ cup sweetened, shredded coconut

1. Preheat oven to 325°F.

2. In a medium bowl, combine condensed milk, egg yolks, lemon zest, and lemon juice with a whisk until blended.

3. Place shells on baking sheets. Fill a zip-lock plastic bag with lemon mixture. Snip off

Belly Tip

Roll the lemon on the counter for a few seconds before juicing it—you'll get more juice out of it. Make sure to remove the zest before you cut the lemon in half to juice it.

a teeny-tiny edge of one of the bottom corners, and fill pastry shells to three-quarters full. Top with coconut. Bake for 7 minutes or until filling is set.

4. Remove from oven and let cool.

5. Loosely cover with plastic wrap (or place in an airtight container), and refrigerate until served. Best served within 4 hours of preparing.

Calories 80; Fat 3 g (Sat 1 g, Mono 0.5 g, Poly 0 g); Cholesterol 48 mg; Protein 2 g; Carbohydrate 12 g; Sugars 7 g; Fiber 0 g; Iron 0 mg; Sodium 246 mg; Calcium 31 mg

Meyer Lemon Granita

Peggy Knickerbocker is a San Francisco–based cookbook author and one of the most creative recipe developers I've worked with. Here's her recipe for a simple, but incredibly refreshing, lemon granita.

This classic Sicilian dessert takes only about 10 minutes to prepare and 2 to 3 hours to freeze. You will need to be around as the granita freezes, as it has to be stirred every half hour or so. Eureka and regular lemons can be used as well, but taste the granita for tartness—you may need to add more sweetener. If you cannot find superfine sugar, place granulated sugar in the bowl of a food processor and pulse for 30 seconds until pulverized.

Prep: 10 minutes

Freeze: 2½ to 3 hours

Makes 6 servings

Momma Must-Have: This is the perfect anti-nausea treat. It's tart and cool, and such a great icy refresher. It's a cool 71 calories.

Zest of 1 lemon, grated

3 cups spring water

2 sprigs fresh mint

½ cup agave syrup, or ⅔ cups of superfine sugar

1 cup fresh meyer lemon juice (about 5 regular meyer lemons)

1. Place the zest, water, mint sprigs, and agave or sugar in a small, heavy saucepan over medium heat. Stir for about 1 minute. Remove from the heat, and allow the syrup to cool slightly in the refrigerator. When chilled, strain out the lemon zest and the mint sprigs.

2. Stir the lemon juice into the chilled syrup. Taste to make sure the mixture is not too tart; if it is, add a little more sugar.

3. Pour the mixture into a 9x13-inch shallow baking dish (metal, ceramic, or glass), so the mixture is about an inch deep. Place in the freezer. Every 30 minutes, stir with a fork, scraping the crystals down from the side of the dish. When the granita is slightly slushy but definitely frozen hard, with small firm granules of ice, it's done. It will take 2 to 3 hours to get to this stage. (The granita may be transferred to an airtight container and stored for a couple of hours before serving.) Remove the granita from the freezer about 10 minutes before serving, so it softens slightly. Serve in dessert bowls or glasses.

Calories 71; Fat 0 g (Sat 0 g, Mono 0 g, Poly 0 g); Cholesterol 0 mg; Protein 0 g; Carbohydrate 22 g; Sugars 19 g; Fiber 0 g; Iron 0 mg; Sodium 1 mg; Calcium 5 mg; Folate 6 mcg

Citrus-Spiked Rice Pudding

Some people have the gene that allows them to make perfect rice. I wasn't born with it, and now I don't have to waste time scraping burned bits from the bottom of my pans. The universe has given me frozen rice, which comes out perfect every time. The other cool thing is that you can just use a little and then reseal the bag and pop it back in the freezer, so there's never an excuse for not having time to make brown rice. If you've got skills with rice or have a rice cooker, by all means, make your own. This recipe also works well with white rice.

Prep: 5 minutes

Cook: 20 minutes

Makes 5 servings

Baby Bonus: Over 10 percent of your bone-building calcium needs for the day.

Momma Must-Have: Three grams of fiber to help you meet your daily goal of 28 to 30 grams.

2 ½ cups frozen brown rice or cooked white or brown rice

1 cup organic 1% milk or vanilla soy milk

2 tablespoons fat-free, sweetened condensed milk

2 teaspoons orange zest

1 teaspoon vanilla extract

½ teaspoon ground cinnamon, plus more for dusting

2 tablespoons maple syrup

½ cup chopped dried apricots, preferably sulfite-free

1. Place the frozen or cooked rice, 1% milk, and sweetened condensed milk in a medium saucepan, and heat over medium heat until simmering, about 5 minutes. Add the zest, vanilla, cinnamon, and maple syrup, and cook an additional 10 minutes, until most of the milk has been absorbed.

2. Stir in the chopped apricots and heat through, about 4 to 5 minutes. Serve warm or cold with a dusting of cinnamon if you'd like.

Calories 204; Fat 2 g (Sat 0.2 g, Mono 0.3 g, Poly 0.3 g); Cholesterol 1 mg; Protein 4 g; Carbohydrate 3 g; Sugars 16 g; Fiber 3 g; Iron 1 mg; Sodium 37 mg; Calcium 111 mg

CREAMY

Carrot Cake Dream Bars

These dreamy little bars are like a cleaned up version of carrot cake. Make them more special with the Basic Cream Cheese Frosting on page 168. Add 2 teaspoons orange zest to the frosting to add some zing.

Prep: 10 minutes

Cook: 30 minutes

Makes 16 squares

Baby Bonus: More than half your vitamin A (from beta-carotene) needs for the day, which means baby's getting a great boost for healthy eyes and skin.

Momma Must-Have: You get to indulge a cakey craving without blowing several hundred calories and up to 30 g of fat on a restaurant-style carrot cake.

1 cup finely shredded carrot

1 egg, whisked

1 tablespoon orange juice

½ cup organic golden raisins

1 tablespoon vanilla extract

½ teaspoon ground cinnamon

½ cup part skim organic ricotta cheese

2 tablespoons butter, melted

¾ cup packed brown sugar

1 cup old-fashioned oats

¼ teaspoon salt

¾ cup whole-wheat flour

1 teaspoon baking powder

1 teaspoon baking soda

⅓ cup chopped walnuts

1. Preheat oven to 350°F.

2. Combine the first seven ingredients (carrot through ricotta cheese) in a large bowl.

3. In a small bowl, stir together the melted butter and the brown sugar. Add to the carrot mixture. Set aside.

4. In a separate medium bowl, combine the dry ingredients (oats through walnuts). Stir the carrot mixture into the dry mixture until fully combined. Do not overmix.

5. Spray an 8x8-inch pan with cooking spray. Pour batter into the pan, and bake for 30 to 33 minutes, or until a toothpick comes out clean. Top with Basic Cream Cheese Frosting if you like. Cut into 16 squares and enjoy.

Calories 215; Fat 6 g (Sat 2 g, Mono 1 g, Poly 2 g) Cholesterol 27 mg; Protein 6 g; Carbohydrate 35 g; Sugars 20 g; Fiber 3 g; Iron 2 mg; Sodium 220 mg; Calcium 68 mg

Basic Cream Cheese Frosting

Prep: 5 minutes

Makes about 15 servings

4 ounces of block-style reduced-fat cream cheese (Neufchatel)

1 teaspoon vanilla extract

1 cup confectioners' sugar

1. Combine all ingredients in a small bowl. Beat on high with an electric mixer until creamy. Spread on top of cupcakes, banana bread, or Carrot Cake Dream Bars.

Calories 57; Fat 2 g (Sat 1 g, Mono 0 g, Poly 0 g); Cholesterol 5 mg; Protein 1 g; Carbohydrate 10 g; Sugars 9 g; Fiber 0 g; Iron 0 mg; Sodium 32 mg; Calcium 5 mg

Oatmeal Brûlée

Half-breakfast, half-dessert, this is so easy to make, it's silly. And there are no blow torches required!

Prep: 3 minutes

Cook: 12 minutes

Makes 4 servings

Baby Bonus: This sweet and healthy treat has 17 percent of your daily calcium needs to help develop strong bones for Baby.

Momma Must-Have: You get to indulge in a decadent-tasting treat while still feeling virtuous that you're eating your heart-healthy oats.

2 cups organic 1% or soy milk

Pinch of salt

1 cup quick-cooking oats

1 tablespoon ground flax seeds

1 cup sliced strawberries or bananas

8 teaspoons brown sugar

1. Add milk and salt to a medium saucepan and bring to a boil over

medium-high heat. Add the oats and turn down to medium. Cook for 10 minutes or until most of the liquid has been absorbed, stirring occasionally. Remove from heat and stir in flax seeds.

2. Turn the broiler on high.

3. Transfer oatmeal to 4 6-ounce ramekins or baking dishes.

4. Layer the sliced berries or bananas on top of the oatmeal. Spoon 2 teaspoons brown sugar on top of each ramekin. Place ramekins on a baking sheet or in a cake pan. Put in the oven on the top rack. Broil for 2 minutes, or until sugar has melted and formed a light crust. Remove from the oven and enjoy.

Calories 185; Fat 4 g (Sat 1 g, Mono 1 g, Poly 1 g); Cholesterol 8 mg; Protein 8 g; Carbohydrate 32 g; Sugars 17 g; Fiber 3 g; Iron 1 mg; Sodium 70 mg; Calcium 173 mg

Mornin' Sunshine Parfait

I love parfaits because they are ridiculously easy to make, but they're pretty enough and girly enough to feel like a special treat. I like making them for weekend guests, or just for myself when I need a little pick-me-up. You'll need parfait glasses or wine glasses for serving.

Prep: 5 minutes

Makes 4 servings

Baby Bonus: It tastes like you're having dessert for breakfast, but it has a healthy 13 g of protein to build Baby's muscles.

Momma Must-Have: Cool, creamy, and delightful. An easy way to entertain for brunch if the in-laws happen to visit.

1½ cups fresh berries, preferably a mix of blueberries, raspberries, and blackberries

2 cups low-fat Greek-style yogurt

½ cup Hippie-Chick Granola (page 180) or your favorite granola

4 teaspoons honey

1. Place about 1 tablespoon of berries in the bottoms of 4 glasses (enough to cover bottom of glass). Then, spoon about ¼ cup of the yogurt into each glass. Top with a little of the granola.

2. Repeat layering the fruit and yogurt. Drizzle 1 teaspoon honey over the yogurt layer, and top each parfait with the remaining granola. Grab a spoon and dig in!

Calories 202; Fat 4 g (Sat 1 g, Mono 0 g, Poly 0 g); Cholesterol 5 mg; Protein 13 g; Carbohydrate 29 g; Sugars 20 g; Fiber 3 g; Iron 1 mg; Sodium 46 mg; Calcium 93 mg

Sweet Baby Bread Pudding

There is nothing like a good bread pudding to satisfy a sweet comfort-food craving. This one is lighter than most, but still rich, creamy, and spot-hitting. The addition of applesauce lets you add less sugar while keeping the pudding plenty sweet. If you don't like currants, or can't find them, dried cherries or golden raisins are great too.

Prep: 10 minutes

Cook: 1 hour (mostly hands-off baking time)

Makes 16 servings

Baby Bonus: About 10 percent of your calcium for the day.

Momma Must-Have: Some restaurant-style bread puddings rack up over 1,000 calories! Dig into the creamy goodness of this one for a fraction of the calories, fat, and sugar.

9 cups cubed ciabatta or other hearty white bread (best if stale)

4 cups organic 1% or soy milk

1½ cups natural sugar

½ cup unsweetened organic applesauce

2 teaspoons vanilla extract

2 large egg whites

2 large eggs

½ teaspoon ground cinnamon

½ cup dried currants

1. Preheat oven to 350°F.

2. Spray a 9x13-inch baking dish with cooking spray. Set aside.

3. Place the cubed bread into a large heatproof bowl.

4. Heat the milk over medium-high heat until bubbling, but not boiling. Pour the hot milk over the bread and allow to soak in.

5. Combine the sugar, applesauce, vanilla, egg whites, eggs, cinnamon, and currants in a medium bowl. Whisk until combined. Add the egg mixture to the bread mixture, and stir until combined. Pour into the prepared pan.

6. Put on the top rack in the oven, and bake for 50 minutes or until bread becomes golden on top and pudding is set.

7. Let sit for about 10 minutes on top of the stove. Then, dig in.

Calories 155; Fat 2 g (Sat 1 g, Mono 1 g, Poly 0 g); Cholesterol 31 mg; Protein 6 g; Carbohydrate 31 g; Sugars 21 g; Fiber 0 g; Iron 1 mg; Sodium 59 mg; Calcium 105 mg

Walnut-Maple Syrup Sauce with Vanilla Ice Cream

Emily Luchetti, the famed pastry chef at San Francisco's Farallon and an award-winning cookbook author, shared this easy, but so delicious, recipe with me. Here's Emily's back-story about how it was created: "My sister-in-law, Lisa, lives in New England. When she was pregnant with her third child, Ethan, she craved maple walnut ice cream. During one of her cravings at my house, I didn't have any. I did have the ingredients to put this five-minute recipe together, which luckily satisfied her."

Prep: 5 to 7 minutes (to toast walnuts)

Cook: 5 minutes

Serves 1

Momma Must-Have: Yes, this recipe comes with a fairly hefty calorie tag, but it's sooo worth it—not only for its creamy decadence, but also for the big calcium bang (20 percent of your daily needs) and the high amount of omega-3 from the walnuts.

¼ cup maple syrup

1 tablespoon cream

2 tablespoons chopped toasted walnuts

1 to 2 scoops of light vanilla ice cream

1. Bring the maple syrup to a boil in a small pot. Boil for about 2 minutes over medium heat until the syrup starts to thicken. (When it does, the boiling bubbles will bubble more slowly.) Remove from heat, and stir in cream. Let cool slightly. The syrup can be made ahead and reheated on top of the stove or in the microwave.

2. Stir in the walnuts. Pour over vanilla ice cream and enjoy!

Calories 434; Fat 15 g (Sat 4 g, Mono 2 g, Poly 7 g, Omega-3 1,350 mg); Cholesterol 16 mg; Protein 6 g; Carbohydrate 74 g; Sugars 64 g; Fiber 1 g; Iron 1 mg; Sodium 62 mg; Calcium 199 mg; Folate 15 mcg

FRUITY

Deconstructed Apple Pie

What's better than apple pie? A dessert that takes just ten minutes to make, can be used in multiple ways, and has just a fraction of apple pie's calories. Before you turn up your nose at the prunes, consider that they'll help keep you regular, and if you chop them finely enough, you can pretend that they're raisins. I love this concoction on its own, but it's also fabulous spooned over vanilla yogurt, as a topping for oatmeal, or as a filling for baked acorn squash. I recommend doubling the recipe; it'll keep in an airtight container in the fridge for about four days.

Prep: 10 minutes

Makes 4 servings

Momma Must-Have: Those grannies have it right—prunes really do help you go to the bathroom. Plus, they're super-rich in anti-oxidants, ranking even higher than blueberries.

1 apple (preferably Fuji or Braeburn), seeded and diced

1 teaspoon orange zest

½ cup walnut halves

1 tablespoon orange juice

2 teaspoons honey (preferably orange blossom)

½ cup chopped pitted prunes

¼ teaspoon ground cinnamon

1. Combine all ingredients in a medium bowl. Enjoy now, or store in an airtight container for up to four days.

Calories 178; Fat 8 g (Sat 1 g, Mono 1 g, Poly 6 g); Cholesterol 1 mg; Protein 3 g; Carbohydrate 26 g; Sugars 15 g; Fiber 3 g; Iron 1 mg; Sodium 3 mg; Calcium 18 mg

Fresh Fruit with Creamy Yo-Co Dip

This is something you can whip up in about five minutes. Use your favorite seasonal fruit, and either drizzle the yogurt mixture over the fruit or dip pieces of fruit into it. The dip will keep in the refrigerator for about three days. Store the fruit separate from the dip to prevent the fruit from turning gross on you.

If you don't have a toaster oven, you may want to skip toasting the flax seeds, since it'll take your oven a while to heat up. Still, the nutty flavor of the toasted seeds is worth the extra time.

Prep: 13 minutes

Makes 6 1-cup servings

Baby Bonus: More than 100 percent of your vitamin C needs for the day, plus omega-3s from the flax seeds for Baby's developing brain.

Super combos:

Winter: Orange and kiwi

Spring: Strawberries and pineapple

Summer: Blueberries and peaches

Fall: Apples, pears, and grapes

2 teaspoons flax seeds

6 cups seasonal fruit, cut into bite-sized pieces

6 ounces creamy-style low-fat organic vanilla yogurt
(such as Wallaby)

¼ cup sweetened coconut flakes

1. Preheat your toaster oven or regular oven to 350°F.

2. Spread the flax seeds in a small pan, and toast for 3 to 5 minutes, stirring halfway through with a wooden spoon. Remove from the oven and allow to cool.

3. Place the fruit in a large bowl.

4. In a small bowl, blend the yogurt with the coconut and the flax seeds.

5. If you're serving a crowd, drizzle the fruit with the yo-co dip and serve in dessert bowls. If you're preparing this as a snack, just dip the fruit into the yo-co, or mix together and enjoy.

Calories 145; Fat 3 g (Sat 2 g, Mono 0 g, Poly 0 g); Cholesterol 2 mg; Protein 3 g; Carbohydrate 33 g; Sugars 22 g; Fiber 4 g; Iron 1 mg; Sodium 34 mg; Calcium 78 mg; Vitamin C 114 mg

Fruity Booty Salad

This is by far not only the prettiest fruit salad I've ever seen, but also the most refreshing. If you're a big fan of ginger, feel free to add more.

Prep: 15 minutes

Makes 4 servings

Baby Bonus: More than 100 percent of your vitamin C for the day, plus beta-carotene for healthy eyes.

Momma Must-Have: With over 500 mg potassium, this recipe will help combat ankle swelling. Ginger and 5 g fiber combine to aid digestion.

2 cups cubed pineapple

1½ cups diced mango

1 small starfruit, sliced

1 kiwi, peeled, sliced and cut into half-moons

1 cup diced ripe papaya

1 banana, sliced

1 tablespoon fresh lemon juice

1 tablespoon fresh lime juice

1 tablespoon fresh grapefruit or orange juice

1 tablespoon honey

½ teaspoon finely chopped fresh ginger

½ teaspoon lime zest

1. Combine all fruit together in a large bowl. Set aside.

2. Add the juices together in a small bowl, and whisk together. Whisk in the honey and remaining ingredients. Pour over the fruit, and refrigerate for at least an hour before serving.

Calories 160; Fat 0.5 g (Sat 0 g, Mono 0 g, Poly 0 g); Cholesterol 0 mg; Protein 2 g; Carbohydrate 41 g; Sugars 30 g; Fiber 5 g; Iron .5 mg; Sodium 4 mg; Calcium 34 mg; Vitamin C 101 mg; Folic Acid 43 mcg; Beta-Carotene 417 mcg; Potassium 503 mg

Peach and Blackberry Crumble

This satisfying dessert can be made with a variety of fruits. Try it with apricots and blueberries, or any combo you have a hankering for. If you're feeling extra decadent, serve the crumble over vanilla ice cream.

Prep: 10 minutes

Cook: 40 minutes

Makes 6 to 8 servings

Baby Bonus: The antioxidant beta-carotene, which is a safe form of vitamin A. It's important for preventing cell damage while your baby is developing.

Momma Must-Have: Beta-carotene is also helpful for warding off colds and is believed to support a woman's reproductive system. This recipe is a sweet, satisfying treat with just 217 calories!

Filling

4 ripe fresh peaches, sliced

1 cup blackberries

1 tablespoon sugar

1 teaspoon fresh lemon juice

¼ teaspoon salt (or just a sprinkle)

Topping

⅓ cup granulated sugar

2 tablespoons brown sugar

½ cup all-purpose flour (or white whole-wheat flour,
such as King Arthur)

¼ teaspoon ground cinnamon

¼ cup regular oats

½ stick butter

1. Preheat oven to 350°F.

2. Combine all the filling ingredients in a medium bowl. Transfer to a 9-inch-round baking dish.

3. Combine all the topping ingredients in a small bowl. Top fruit with oat topping.

4. Bake for 40 minutes, or until topping is golden and fruit is oozy. Try to wait 10 minutes for it to cool down before eating. If not, try not to burn your tongue!

Calories 217; Fat 8 g (Sat 5 g, Mono 2 g, Poly 0.5 g); Cholesterol 20 mg; Protein 2 g; Carbohydrate 36 g; Sugars 24 g; Fiber 3 g; Iron 1 mg; Sodium 100 mg; Calcium 20 mg; Folate 10 mcg; Beta-Carotene 151 mcg

Salty/Sweet

Baby on Board Banana Bread

The first time I made this I completely left out the sugar (blame it on pregnancy fog), but it actually still turned out really nicely. The overripe bananas give it a ton of natural sweetness, and you can always drizzle some honey on top. Of course, if you prefer it sweeter, add the brown sugar.

Prep: 15 minutes

Cook: 40 minutes

Makes 8 servings

Momma Must-Have: A slice of regular banana bread usually has only half as much fiber as this version and only a scant amount of calcium. So enjoy your slice of the sweet stuff, knowing that it's actually quite good for you.

1 cup whole-wheat flour

½ cup all-purpose flour

1 teaspoon baking soda

1 tablespoon dry milk powder

⅛ teaspoon salt

½ cup brown sugar (optional)

1½ tablespoons ground flax seed

1 egg

½ cup organic 1% milk

2 tablespoons unsalted butter, melted

¼ cup organic low-fat vanilla yogurt

½ teaspoon vanilla extract

3 ripe bananas (about 2 cups)

1 cup chopped almonds

1. Preheat oven to 350°F. Coat an 8½ x 4½-inch pan with cooking spray.

2. Mix the dry ingredients (flours, baking soda, dry milk powder, salt, brown sugar, and ground flax seed) together in a medium bowl.

3. In a separate bowl, whisk the egg. To the egg, add the milk, melted butter, yogurt, and vanilla. Whisk until combined, and mash in the bananas.

4. Stir the wet ingredients into the dry until just incorporated. Do not overmix (or air bubbles will form).

5. Transfer batter to the prepared pan. Top with the chopped almonds, and bake for 40 minutes, or until golden brown. Cool for 10 minutes, then serve.

Calories 226; Fat 4 g (Sat 1 g, Mono 0 g, Poly 0.5 g); Cholesterol 28 mg; Protein 6 g; Carbohydrate 43 g; Sugars 21 g; Fiber 4 g; Iron 1 mg; Sodium 291 mg; Calcium 83 mg; Folate 18 mcg; Potassium 202 mg

Hippie-Chick Granola

This packed-full-of-goodies granola is wickedly tasty, but has all the goodness you'd expect from your local health food co-op. It's great as a topper for less tasty cereal, and it's perfect for adding a bit of crunch to yogurt or ice cream. Pack some up for on-the-go treats in snack-size zip-lock bags.

Prep: 8 minutes

Cook: 23 minutes

Makes 6 cups of granola (12 ⅓-cup servings)

Momma Must-Have: Skip the high-fructose corn syrup, tropical oils, and preservatives that you'll find in many commercial brands of granola. This one gives you 3 g fiber per serving, plus heart-healthy almonds and pumpkin seeds.

½ cup oat bran flakes

2 cups old-fashioned oats

¼ cup slivered almonds

¼ cup roasted pumpkin seeds

¼ cup dried currants or raisins

¼ cup dried cranberries

½ cup dried tart cherries

¼ cup flax seeds

½ cup honey

⅓ cup (5 tablespoons) unsalted butter, melted

1. Preheat oven to 350°F. Coat a baking sheet or jelly roll pan with cooking spray; set aside.

2. In a large mixing bowl, combine the bran flakes, oats, almonds, pumpkin seeds, currants, cranberries, cherries, and flax seeds. Set aside.

3. In a small bowl, combine the honey and melted butter, and pour over the oat and fruit mixture. Stir with a wooden spoon until combined.

4. Spread mixture onto the prepared pan, and bake for 23 minutes or until golden. Cool on the pan, and break into pieces

with a spatula. Store in an airtight container (I like a glass jar) for up to a week.

Calories 228; Fat 10 g (Sat 4 g, Mono 1 g, Poly 0 g); Cholesterol 13 mg; Protein 5 g; Carbohydrate 30 g; Sugars 16 g; Fiber 3 g; Iron 1 mg; Sodium 7 mg; Calcium 22 mg; Folate 3 mcg; Beta-Carotene 104 mcg; Potassium 21 mg

Morning, Noon, and Night Nut Clusters

Pastry chef David Guas will always have a special place in my heart because he made our wedding cake. He's also incredibly good at creating the perfect treat to suit any craving. That's exactly what he did for his wife, Simone, when she wanted something salty-sweet and crunchy during her second pregnancy. I can attest that these little nuggets are addictive. Bake these on silicone mats if you have them.

Prep: 15 minutes

Cook: 20 minutes

Makes about 32 clusters

Momma Must-Have: These are only 60 calories a pop, but I can't guarantee you'll eat only one. These low-sugar, high-protein bites are super-satisfying and so easy to make.

1 cup almonds, chopped

1 cup cashews, roughly chopped

¼ cup light brown sugar, packed

2 tablespoons honey

1 egg white

½ teaspoon salt

⅓ cup dried cherries (or cranberries, currants, raisins), chopped

1. Preheat oven to 325°F.

2. Toast nuts on a baking sheet lined with parchment paper for 10 to 15 minutes or until golden brown. Stir the nuts halfway through for even browning. Remove from the oven and cool. Keep the oven set at 325°F.

3. In a large stainless steel mixing bowl, vigorously whisk the sugar, honey, and egg white together until foamy, approximately 1 minute. Sprinkle in the salt, cherries, and toasted cooled nuts, and stir with a rubber spatula until fully combined.

4. Line two baking sheets with parchment paper, and spray parchment with cooking spray (unless using silicone mats). Using a small spoon, portion the mix onto the parchment-lined baking sheets in small clusters (just a bit larger than a quarter). Bake the clusters for 15 to 20 minutes or until they are light amber and no longer sticky to the touch. Remove from the oven, and allow to cool for 20 to 30 minutes before eating. Store in an airtight container at room temperature for up to 10 days. If they begin to get a little soft, you can bake them again at 275°F for 8 to 10 minutes. But I doubt they'll last that long!

Calories 60; Fat 4 g (Sat 0.5 g, Mono 2 g, Poly 1 g); Cholesterol 0 mg; Protein 2 g; Carbohydrate 6 g; Sugars 4 g; Fiber 1 g; Iron 0.5 mg; Sodium 39 mg; Calcium 12 mg; Folate 4 mcg; Potassium 56 mg

Courtesy of David Guas, Chef, Author, Consultant, Damgoodsweet Consulting Group, LLC

Oh, Baby! Breakfast Cookies

You know those mornings—the kind where you can barely stomach a glass of water—and getting anything to stay down is a challenge. Even on those days, you know you need to get something in your belly. This healthy cookie does the trick, and they're equally good in the afternoon, too. Dates really make the texture nice and chewy, but raisins work too.

Prep: 10 minutes

Cook: 12 minutes

Makes 30 cookies

Momma Must-Have: These little jewels let you satisfy your sweet tooth for less than 100 calories, but they're so packed with tasty ingredients that it's hard to believe. Whole oats and almonds help boost the fiber and heart-healthiness of these cookies, while dates add a ton of natural sweetness and chewiness.

6 tablespoons unsalted butter

¾ cup packed brown sugar

⅓ cup all-purpose flour

⅓ cup whole-wheat flour

¾ teaspoon baking soda

1½ cups regular oats

½ teaspoon salt

1 egg

1 teaspoon vanilla extract

½ cup chopped pitted dates

¼ cup chopped almonds

¼ cup sweetened coconut

¼ cup dried cherries

1. Preheat oven to 350°F. Lightly spray two baking sheets with cooking spray, or cover sheets with silicone baking mats.

2. Melt the butter in a small saucepan over low heat.

3. Remove the saucepan from heat, and add the brown sugar, stirring until smooth.

4. Combine the dry ingredients—the flours, baking soda, oats, and salt—in a medium bowl.

5. Add the butter-sugar mixture to the dry ingredients.

6. Whisk the egg gently in a small bowl, and add to the mixture, along with the vanilla. Add the dates, almonds, coconut, and cherries, and mix well.

7. Spoon the mixture by tablespoonfuls onto the prepared pans. Bake for 12 minutes or until tops are lightly golden and dry to the touch. Remove from the oven, and allow to cool slightly. Attempt to eat just one at a time!

Calories 90; Fat 4 g (Sat 2 g, Mono 0.5 g, Poly 0 g); Cholesterol 13 mg; Protein 1.5 g; Carbohydrate 14 g; Sugars 8 g; Fiber 1 g; Iron 0.5 mg; Sodium 77 mg; Calcium 12 mg; Folate 4 mcg; Potassium 64 mg

MEATY

POULTRY, RED MEAT, PORK

Chicken Pot Pie

Nothing says comfort quite like a chicken pot pie. The creamy chicken and veggies peeking out from under a flaky crust gets me every time. My friend Tanya couldn't get enough pot pie during her second pregnancy—it was the only thing that helped calm her stomach.

This recipe takes much less time than most because you cook the chicken before putting the pie in the oven, and you use foolproof refrigerated dough. Save even more time and buy chicken tenders instead of whole chicken breasts.

Prep: 10 minutes

Cook: 56 minutes

Makes 6 servings

Baby Bonus: With 23 g protein per serving, this recipe helps form Baby's growing body.

Momma Must-Have: Each serving has 10 percent of your daily iron needs to keep you and Baby going strong. When you're not feeling like eating your veggies, this is a great way to sneak some in.

1 tablespoon olive oil, plus 1 teaspoon

½ yellow onion, chopped (about 1 cup)

½ cup diced celery

1 pound organic or natural chicken breast halves,
cut into bite-sized pieces

¼ teaspoon salt

¼ teaspoon freshly ground pepper

2 tablespoons all-purpose flour

2 cups reduced sodium chicken broth

¼ teaspoon freshly ground nutmeg

1 1-pound bag frozen organic mixed vegetables,
defrosted and drained

1½ 8-ounce packages refrigerated,
reduced-fat refrigerated crescent-roll dough (such as Pillsbury)

1. Preheat oven to 350°F.

2. Heat 1 tablespoon oil in a large skillet over medium-high heat. Add the onion and celery, and cook until onion is translucent and slightly golden, about 4 minutes.

3. Turn heat down to medium, add chicken to the pan, and season with salt and pepper. Cook for 5 minutes, turn the pieces of chicken, and cook for another 5 minutes, or until chicken is cooked through and reaches an internal temperature of 165°F. Transfer chicken to a plate.

4. In the same pan, add the remaining teaspoon of oil, and heat over medium heat. Add the flour, and stir until pasty, about 2 minutes. Add the broth, and stir until mixture becomes smooth. Stir in the nutmeg. Increase heat and bring to a boil; turn down heat and simmer 15 minutes, until mixture thickens.

5. Add the chicken and defrosted mixed vegetables back to the pan, and stir until well combined. Transfer to a 9-inch pie dish.

6. Lay the crescent-roll dough over the top of the dish in an overlapping pattern until the filling is entirely covered. Put in the

oven, and bake for 25 minutes, or until crust is golden and crisp. Let sit for about 10 minutes, and then serve.

Calories 386; Fat 14.5 g (Sat 3 g, Mono 3 g, Poly 1 g); Cholesterol 42 mg; Protein 23 g; Carbohydrate 38 g; Sugars 9 g; Fiber 4 g; Iron 3 mg; Sodium 607 mg; Calcium 36 mg; Folate 25 mcg; Beta-Carotene 160 mcg

Koto Kapama (Cinnamon-Stewed Chicken)

Cat Cora is a serious chef. In fact, she's the first woman ever to kick ass on Iron Chef. Cat's Greek heritage inspired this hearty dish when her partner was expecting. Cooking the chicken with the skin on helps to keep it moist and flavorful, but feel free to remove it once it's done cooking (the nutritional analysis was calculated without the skin).

Here are Cat's own thoughts: "This is a warm, comforting, and flavorful dish that Jennifer and I both love to eat. It's low in fat because I use olive oil instead of butter or cream, and Jennifer always craved its heartiness when she was pregnant. We still prepare this for dinner often—it is definitely one of our all-time favorites."

Note: Ask your butcher to cut the chicken into pieces for you. Post-pregnancy, try adding ½ cup dry white wine to the pan after you've sautéed the onions.

Prep: 10 minutes

Cook: 72 minutes

Makes 6 servings

Baby Bonus: One serving nearly knocks out your protein needs for the day and helps Junior grow strong. And 10 percent of your iron requirement helps ensure a strong blood supply.

Momma Must-Have: Since this recipe satisfies almost 20 percent of your zinc needs, it'll keep your immune system humming, and you also get tons of potassium to help prevent muscle cramps.

1 chicken (2½ to 3 pounds), cut into eight pieces

1 teaspoon ground cinnamon

2 teaspoons kosher salt

1 teaspoon freshly ground black pepper

1½ tablespoons extra-virgin olive oil

5 cloves garlic, minced and divided

2 medium yellow onions, coarsely chopped

1 cup water

1 cup chicken stock

1 6-ounce can tomato paste

1 tablespoon fresh oregano, chopped

1. Pat the chicken dry with paper towels. Mix the cinnamon, kosher salt, and pepper in a small bowl. Rub the spice mix all over the chicken pieces.

2. Heat the olive oil in a large, deep skillet over high heat (a 12-inch skillet with sides about 2½ to 3 inches high will allow you to brown all the chicken at once). Add the chicken to the oil, and brown for about four to five minutes on each side, until well browned all over. Transfer chicken to a plate.

3. Lower the heat to medium-high, and add the onions and 3 minced cloves of garlic. Cook for about 3 minutes, stirring constantly, until the onions have softened and are a rich golden brown.

4. Return the chicken to the pan, and add the water, chicken stock, tomato paste, oregano, and remaining garlic cloves. The liquid should cover the chicken about three-quarters of the way. Cover the pot and

simmer over low heat for about 1 hour, until the chicken is tender and thoroughly cooked. Season the finished sauce with kosher salt and pepper to taste. Serve over a bed of quinoa or another favorite grain.

Calories 334; Fat 7 g (Sat 1 g, Mono 3 g, Poly 1 g); Cholesterol 132 mg; Protein 55 g; Carbohydrate 12 g; Sugars 6 g; Fiber 3 g; Iron 3 mg; Sodium 789 mg; Calcium 64 mg; Folate 23 mcg; Beta-Carotene 266 mcg; Potassium 959 mg; Zinc 2 mg

Courtesy of Cat Cora's Kitchen

Lemony Chicken with Capers

When you want a dish with a nice tang to it, this one really hits the spot. The lemon juice and capers give it a bright, salty balance.

Prep: 12 minutes

Cook: 7 minutes

Makes 4 servings

Momma Must-Have: This is a great thing to make when you just don't feel like cooking, because it takes less than 20 minutes. Knock out ⅓ of your protein for the day and have calories to spare for dessert.

½ cup all-purpose flour (you won't use all of it)

¼ teaspoon salt

¼ teaspoon pepper

½ teaspoon herbs de Provence

1 pound organic or natural chicken cutlets

1 tablespoon olive oil

2 tablespoons fresh lemon juice

½ cup chicken broth

2 tablespoons capers, drained

1. Combine the flour, salt, pepper, and herbs de Provence in a small bowl. Dredge the chicken cutlets in the flour mixture, and transfer to a plate.

2. Heat the oil in a large nonstick skillet over medium-high heat. Add the chicken cutlets to the pan, and cook for 4 minutes per side, or until golden brown. Transfer to a clean plate, and cover with foil.

3. To the same skillet, add the lemon juice, chicken broth, and capers. Use a spatula to scrape up any browned bits in the pan. Cook for 3 minutes. Pour sauce over chicken and serve. This is great with brown rice and sautéed spinach.

Calories 187; Fat 5 g (Sat 1 g, Mono 3 g, Poly 1 g); Cholesterol 66 mg; Protein 27 g; Carbohydrate 7 g; Sugars 1 g; Fiber 0.5 g; Iron 1 mg; Sodium 418 mg; Calcium 18 mg; Folate 17 mcg

Mini Meatballs with Kale and Orecchiette

If you haven't tried ground bison—buffalo—yet, give it a chance. The flavor is really good, and these days you can find it in most grocery stores. It's an even richer source of zinc, iron, and vitamin B_{12} than beef is, plus it's much lower in fat. Ground lamb is also excellent in this recipe. I know the ingredient list on this one is kind of scary-long, but it's a nutrient powerhouse that's totally worth it. This recipe has a broth-like consistency, so serve it with some nice crusty bread to sop up all the tasty juices.

Prep: 20 minutes

Cook: 33 minutes

Makes 6 servings

Baby Bonus: Baby's in for a treat. You get mega-iron in this one from the bison plus the kale. You also knock out your beta-carotene needs, and more than half of your B_{12} to keep baby's nerve cells and red blood cells healthy.

Momma Must-Have: Over 20 percent of your daily folate—important for baby's spinal development, and it may also be tied to your mental health.

1 cup finely chopped red onion

2 cloves garlic, minced

½ cup panko (Japanese breadcrumbs)

2 tablespoons plain, low-fat Greek-style yogurt

1 pound ground bison (buffalo) or lamb

1 egg, beaten

¼ cup chopped flat-leaf parsley

1 teaspoon kosher salt, divided

¼ teaspoon freshly ground black pepper

¼ teaspoon ground allspice

¾ teaspoon Worcestershire sauce

1½ tablespoons olive oil

10-ounce package of dried orecchiette (ear-shaped pasta), such as De Cecco brand

1¼ cups organic chicken broth, divided

1 bunch kale (5 cups), chopped, leaves still wet

¼ teaspoon crushed red pepper

2 tablespoons grated Parmesan, for serving

1. Place a large pot of water on the stove to boil. Preheat oven to 350°F.

2. Combine the first 7 ingredients (red onion through parsley) in a large bowl. Add in ½ teaspoon kosher salt, the pepper, allspice, and Worcestershire sauce. Stir with a spatula until well combined.

3. Place a sheet of parchment paper on a baking sheet or large platter. Spoon out the bison mixture using a tablespoon, and shape into meatballs by rolling mixture between your (clean!) hands. Set meatballs on lined baking sheet as you make them.

4. Heat the olive oil in a large skillet over medium-high heat. Working in batches (unless you have a really big pan), add the meatballs in an even layer, and cook on each side for 5 minutes, or until evenly browned. Transfer the meatballs to a baking dish, and place in the preheated oven for 10 minutes to finish cooking.

5. Cook the orecchiette, once the water starts boiling, according to package directions. Drain.

5. Using the same skillet (don't clean it), add ¼ cup of the chicken broth and use a spatula to scrape up the browned bits from the pan. Add the chopped kale, cover, and heat over medium-high for about 8 minutes or until wilted. Sprinkle the kale with the pepper flakes, ¼ teaspoon of the remaining salt, and add the remaining 1 cup chicken broth. Bring to a simmer for 5 minutes.

6. Combine the meatballs, kale, and any remaining liquid in a large bowl with the orecchiette. Add the remaining salt and stir well. Sprinkle with the Parmesan, and serve hot.

Calories 462; Fat 19 g (Sat 7 g, Mono 7 g, Poly 1 g); Cholesterol 94 mg; Protein 26 g; Carbohydrate 49 g; Sugars 4 g; Fiber 4 g; Iron 5 mg; Sodium 588 mg; Calcium 156 mg; Folate 135 mcg; Beta-Carotene 5295 mcg; Potassium 611 mg; Vitamin B$_{12}$ 1.35 mcg; Zinc 4 mg

Momma's Meatloaf

Save time and get bagged shredded carrots. I prefer brown eggs, and if you can find the ones enhanced with omega-3s, go for 'em.

Prep: 10 minutes

Cook: 70 minutes

Makes 6 servings

Baby Bonus: Calcium for Baby's growing bones and teeth (yep, they're already forming), plus 22 grams of protein to help her whole body grow.

Momma Must-Have: More than 10 percent of your daily iron (in an easy-to-absorb form) to help meet your increased needs. Plus, this is some serious comfort food without the guilt!

Meatloaf

1 cup beef stock, divided

1 medium onion, minced

1½ cups unseasoned whole-wheat panko or regular breadcrumbs

¼ to ½ cup grated Parmesan cheese, depending on preference

½ cup shredded carrot

½ cup chopped fresh flat-leaf parsley

1 teaspoon whole-grain Dijon mustard

1 pound ground bison

2 eggs, whisked

2 teaspoons salt

¼ teaspoon black pepper

Sauce

¼ cup apple cider vinegar

¼ cup packed brown sugar

3 tablespoons tomato paste

2 tablespoons ketchup

1 tablespoon Worcestershire sauce

1. Preheat oven to 350°F. Spray an 8½ x 4¼ x 2¾-inch nonstick loaf pan with cooking spray and set aside.

2. Add half the stock to a medium pan, and heat over medium-high heat. Add the onion, and sauté until translucent, about 5 minutes. Set aside and allow to cool. (If you add the hot onion to the egg-meat mixture too quickly, the eggs will begin to cook.)

3. Combine the onions and all the remaining meatloaf ingredients in a large mixing bowl. Transfer to the prepared loaf pan.

4. Bake for 45 minutes. Meanwhile, combine the sauce ingredients (apple cider vinegar, brown sugar, tomato paste, ketchup, and Worcestershire sauce) in a small bowl.

5. Remove the meatloaf from the oven, and spread sauce on top with a spatula. Return to oven.

6. Bake for an additional 20 minutes, until sauce appears thick and bubbly. Remove from oven, and allow to cool slightly before slicing. Serve warm.

Calories 352; Fat 15 g (Sat 6 g, Mono 5 g, Poly 1 g); Cholesterol 128 mg; Protein 22 g; Carbohydrate 33 g; Sugars 14 g; Fiber 2 g; Iron 3 mg; Sodium 610 mg; Calcium 102 mg; Folate 19 mcg

Pork Chops with Asparagus and Morels

This recipe comes from my friend, San Francisco-based culinary instructor Joanne Weir. Making perfect use of spring ingredients, this dish combines morel mushrooms and asparagus for an earthy-nutty flavor. Joanne suggests brining the chops for an additional bit of juiciness. If morels are super-expensive, just buy a few and throw them in with regular mushrooms for a flavor boost. This dish has a nice "wow" factor on the plate but is easy to make, so it's perfect for those times when you want to impress.

Prep: 15 minutes

Cook: 28 minutes

Stand: 20 minutes

Makes 6 servings

Baby Bonus: Baby gets 20 percent of the choline she needs for brain development and a good memory down the road.

Momma Must-Have: Knock out half of your daily protein requirements with one serving.

For brining (optional): Wash the pork chops and place in a big bowl. For each 1 cup of water, dissolve 1 tablespoon kosher salt. Completely submerge the pork chops in the salted water, and let sit in the refrigerator for 1 hour. Remove from the refrigerator, drain, and pat dry.

¼ ounce dried morel mushrooms
(or other dried wild mushrooms)

6 center-cut pork chops, each about 4 to 6 ounces and
1 inch thick, trimmed of excess fat

Kosher salt

Freshly ground black pepper

¾ pound asparagus, ends trimmed, cut into 1½-inch pieces

2 tablespoons extra-virgin olive oil, divided

1½ cups chicken stock

½ pound fresh morel mushrooms
(or other wild mushrooms), halved

1 teaspoon chopped fresh thyme

Thyme sprigs, for garnish

1. Bring a saucepan of salted water to a boil. Meanwhile, in a small bowl, combine ½ cup boiling water and the dried morels. Let cool to room temperature, about 20 minutes.

2. Line a strainer with cheesecloth, and drain the mushrooms, reserving the liquid. Chop the mushrooms and set aside. (Tip: If you don't have cheesecloth, you can use a white paper towel in a pinch.)

3. When the water is boiling, add the asparagus and cook until tender yet crisp, 3 to 5 minutes. Drain and reserve.

4. In a frying pan large enough to hold the chops in a single layer without crowding, warm 1 tablespoon of the olive oil over medium heat. Add the pork chops and cook, uncovered, for 5 minutes. Turn them over and season with salt and pepper. Reduce the heat to medium-low and continue to cook, uncovered, turning occasionally, until golden and firm to the touch, about 8 to 9 minutes longer. Remove from the pan, place on a warm platter, and cover with aluminum foil.

5. Pour the chicken stock into a saucepan, and boil rapidly to reduce by half. Set aside.

6. In the frying pan used to cook the pork chops, heat the remaining 1 tablespoon olive oil over medium-high heat. Add the fresh and reserved dried morels, and cook until the fresh mushrooms are tender, 3 to 4 minutes. Remove the mushrooms from the

pan, and reserve with the pork. Turn the heat to high, add the chicken stock, thyme, and mushroom liquid, and reduce until it thickens slightly, 3 to 5 minutes. Add the reserved asparagus, and warm for 1 minute.

7. Place the pork chops on individual plates, and divide the sauce, asparagus, and mushrooms over the top. Garnish with thyme sprigs and serve.

Reprinted with permission from *Wine Country Cooking* by Joanne Weir. Copyright 1999, 2008 by Joanne Weir, Ten Speed Press, Berkeley, CA. www.tenspeed.com.

Calories 277; Fat 12 g (Sat 3 g, Mono 7 g, Poly 2 g); Cholesterol 89 mg; Protein 34 g; Carbohydrate 6 g; Sugars 2 g; Fiber 3 g; Iron 1 mg; Sodium 398 mg; Calcium 19 mg

Tuscan Turkey Burgers

Ground turkey is pretty blah on its own, but you can use it as a neutral palette and take it in various flavor directions. Instead of this Tuscan version, try using feta and black olives for a Greek-style burger (great with lamb), or cilantro and ground chili pepper for a Mexican kick.

Prep: 5 minutes

Cook: 12 minutes

Makes 4 to 5 servings

Baby Bonus: A whopping 34 percent of the calcium you need for the day helps boost Baby's growing bones. You'll also get 40 percent of your protein requirement, practically knocking out your baby-building needs for the day (60 g).

Momma Must-Have: Iron, fiber, and lots of flavor. If you're feeling a little bloated, skip the cheese and bun—they both have quite a bit of sodium.

Cooking tips: The burgers can be made in a nonstick skillet or grill pan, but of course they'd also be great cooked on a grill. If they're not up to 165°F when you first take their temperature, make sure to wash the meat thermometer with soapy water before re-inserting it into the burger.

1 pound 99 percent fat-free ground turkey breast

¼ cup chopped flat-leaf parsley

1 large clove garlic, minced

1 tablespoon shredded Parmesan cheese

½ teaspoon fresh or ¼ teaspoon dried thyme leaves

2 teaspoons aged balsamic vinegar

¼ teaspoon kosher salt

¼ teaspoon pepper

4 1-ounce slices asiago cheese

1 cup arugula

4 whole-wheat buns

1. Spray a large, nonstick skillet or grill pan with cooking spray. Set on burner.

2. In a large bowl, mix the turkey, parsley, garlic, Parmesan cheese, thyme, balsamic vinegar, salt, and pepper with clean hands (if this grosses you out, ask someone else to do this step). Using a ½-cup measure, form burgers into patties and transfer to a plate. Wash your hands.

3. Heat the skillet over high heat, and add burgers to skillet (do not reuse the plate that held the raw burgers). Cook on each side 5 to 6 minutes, slightly flattening with a spatula. Using a meat thermometer, check that the internal temperature reaches 165°F.

4. Top each burger with a slice of the asiago cheese, and allow to melt, about 2 minutes. Toast the buns while the cheese is melting.

5. Use a spatula to place each burger on a bun. Top with ¼ cup arugula and the condiments of your choice. Serve hot.

Calories 377; Fat 15 g (Sat 7 g, Mono 2 g, Poly 1 g); Cholesterol 76 mg; Protein 40 g; Carbohydrate 26 g; Sugars 4 g; Fiber 4 g; Iron 3 mg; Sodium 873 mg; Calcium 336 mg; Folate 26 mcg; Beta-Carotene 294 mcg; Biotin 3 mcg; Zinc 1 mg

SEAFOOD

Baked Mediterranean Tilapia

Even my husband, who isn't a big fan of fish, said he'd eat it all the time if it was prepared like this. In addition to baking the packets in the oven, you can also cook them on the grill. Cooking in parchment steams the food inside, leaving it juicy and perfectly cooked. It's a great low-fat cooking method because you don't need to add much oil. It also works for thinly cut vegetables, seafood, and even chicken cutlets.

Prep: 5 minutes

Cook: 15 minutes

Makes 2 servings (can easily be made for more)

Baby Bonus: Baby nets 310 mg (200 is the recommendation) of omega-3 for her brain development.

Momma Must-Have: You pack in 45 grams of protein in a very slim (less than 300 calories) package. Plus, it's a cinch to make!

2 6-ounce tilapia fillets

4 slices lemon

8 slices garlic (about 1 large clove)

6 kalamata olives, halved

1 to 2 teaspoons fresh thyme leaves

2 teaspoons extra-virgin olive oil

Salt and pepper

1. Preheat oven to 400°F.

2. Tear off two large squares of parchment paper (you can also use foil, but it's not as pretty). Fold in half.

3. Open the folded squares, and on half of each piece of parchment, place a piece of tilapia. On each fillet, add the following: 2 slices lemon, 4 slices garlic, 6 olive halves, a bit of fresh thyme, 1 teaspoon extra-virgin olive oil, and a sprinkle of salt and pepper. Fold the top of the parchment over, and roll up the sides tightly, making small crimps in the paper.

4. Place both packets on a baking sheet, and bake for 15 to 20 minutes, until the fish is opaque and flakes easily. Note: Be careful when opening the packets. Snip a corner with a pair of kitchen shears and allow some steam to release. After the steam has released, you can either transfer the tilapia directly to plates or place the packets onto plates and serve.

Calories 294; Fat 12 g (Sat 3 g, Mono 7 g, Poly 2 g, Omega-3 310 mg); Cholesterol 97 mg; Protein 45 g; Carbohydrate 2 g; Sugars 0 g; Fiber 0 g; Iron 1 mg; Sodium 425 mg; Calcium 35 mg; Folate 10 mcg

Ginger-Glazed Salmon

Recent studies have found that omega-3 fatty acids are great for just about everything, from keeping your skin and heart healthy to staving off depression. Most importantly for you right now is the news that eating enough seafood while you're pregnant (of course avoiding the no-no list of fish on page 58) actually helps make Junior smarter. Babies whose moms had eaten at least 340 grams (about 12 ounces) of seafood a week had higher scores on tests for motor skills, social development, and communication. So Mom was right—again: Fish is brain food.

Prep: 2 minutes

Cook: 14 minutes

Makes 2 servings

Baby Bonus: Mega amounts of omega-3 fatty acids for Baby's healthy brain development and protein for Baby's growing body.

Momma Must-Have: Stomach-settling ginger and a recipe that's quick enough for busy weeknights.

2 teaspoons olive oil

1 shallot, minced

1 teaspoon fish sauce

1 teaspoon low-sodium soy sauce

1 to 2 teaspoons ginger juice (such as the Ginger People's, available at Whole Foods) or grated fresh ginger

2 4-ounce salmon fillets, skin removed

1 teaspoon honey

1. Heat oil in a sauté pan over medium-high heat.

2. Add shallot, and cook until golden, about 1 minute.

3. Add fish sauce, soy sauce, and ginger juice or grated ginger to pan; stir.

4. Add fish to pan, and cook for 6 minutes per side, or until opaque in the middle. Transfer salmon to 2 serving plates.

5. Add honey to pan, allow sauce to thicken slightly, 1 to 2 minutes, and drizzle over fish. Serve hot with Sesame-Ginger Green
Beans (page 247) or steamed baby bok choy.

Calories 243; Fat 8 g (Sat 1 g, Mono 4 g, Poly 2 g, Omega-3 1,960 mg); Cholesterol 72
mg; Protein 26 g; Carbohydrate 5 g; Sugars 3 g; Fiber 0 g; Iron 1 mg; Sodium 378 mg;
Calcium 20 mg; Folate 34 mcg

Shrimp with Peas and Pesto

This is a great freezer-and-pantry dish that's perfect for busy weeknights. The key ingredient is really the pesto, so pick a brand you've
used before and like.

Prep: 5 minutes

Cook: 20 minutes

Makes 4 servings

Baby Bonus: As far as nutrients go, this recipe is the bomb. Not
only does it meet your omega-3 needs for the day, but if you use a
calcium-fortified pasta, you'll also get half the calcium you need for
the day. Did I mention that it has over a quarter of your folate, too?

Momma Must-Have: Check it out—you get 11 g fiber in one serving! And since shrimp is such a great source of iron, you get 20
percent of what you need for the day.

1 14.5-ounce box whole-grain rotini with extra calcium
and fiber (such as Ronzoni Smart Taste)

2 cups frozen peas

2 teaspoons olive oil

1 16-ounce bag peeled, deveined frozen shrimp, defrosted

¼ cup plus 1 tablespoon bottled pesto

1 6 ½-ounce jar marinated artichoke hearts, drained and chopped

2 tablespoons chopped flat-leaf parsley

1. Place a large pot of water on the stove to boil.

2. Once the water is boiling, cook pasta according to package directions. With 2 minutes of cooking time remaining, add the peas to the cooking water. Drain, reserving ½ cup of the cooking liquid.

3. Heat the oil in a large skillet (12-inch size is ideal) over medium-high heat. Add the shrimp and heat through, about 4 minutes. Add the cooked pasta and peas to the shrimp, and cook an additional 2 minutes. Stir in the pesto and artichoke hearts. Add the reserved cooking liquid and stir again.

4. Divide the pasta into 4 bowls, and sprinkle equal amounts of the parsley on top. Serve while hot.

Calories 490; Fat 16 g (Sat 3 g, Mono 7 g, Poly 2 g, Omega-3 650 mg); Cholesterol 179 mg; Protein 36 g; Carbohydrate 57 g; Sugars 1 g; Fiber 11 g; Iron 6 mg; Sodium 378 mg; Calcium 508 mg; Folate 154 mcg; Beta-Carotene 95 mcg

VEGETARIAN

Everything but the Kitchen Sink Frittata

You'll want to master the frittata now, because it'll save you from resorting to take-out pizza and fast food once your little one is big enough for grown-up fare. All you really need to have on hand are eggs and some cheese that can be grated. The rest of the ingredients will magically come from your fridge and pantry, whether it's leftover chicken breasts and pasta, or a bottle of sun-dried tomatoes that have been languishing in the pantry. Oh, and a good nonstick pan that can go in the oven really helps too. Try replacing the potatoes in this recipe with an equal amount of cooked spaghetti.

Prep: 10 minutes

Cook: 18 minutes

Makes 6 servings

Baby Bonus: The eggs provide a healthy dose of choline for Baby's brain health and a ton of beta-carotene for her developing eyes.

Momma Must-Have: You get a bit of all the good stuff (iron, folate, potassium), plus a recipe you're likely to make again and again.

1 tablespoon olive oil

1 small onion, diced

5-ounce package of fresh baby spinach

2 cups cooked diced potatoes, or mashed potatoes

1 teaspoon chopped fresh rosemary, or any other fresh herb you like

3 eggs

3 egg whites

¼ teaspoon salt

¼ teaspoon pepper

2 tablespoons shredded aged cheddar

1. Preheat oven to 350°F.

2. Heat the oil over medium-high heat in a 10- to 12-inch non-stick skillet with a heatproof handle. Add the onion, and cook for about 2 minutes, until translucent. Add the spinach, and sauté for 1 minute. Add the cooked potatoes to the pan (if using mashed potatoes, press down into pan with the back of a spatula) along with the rosemary, and cook for an additional 5 minutes, until potatoes start to become golden.

3. Meanwhile, whisk the eggs and egg whites together in a medium bowl, adding the salt and pepper. Pour into the pan over the potatoes, tilting the pan a bit to distribute the eggs. Cook for about 5 minutes, until edges look dry but top looks wet.

4. Sprinkle the cheese over the top of the frittata, and put in the oven for 5 minutes, or until the top is fully cooked and the cheese has melted.

Calories 197; Fat 8 g (Sat 2 g, Mono 2.5 g, Poly 1 g); Cholesterol 165 mg; Protein 11 g; Carbohydrate 21 g; Sugars 3 g; Fiber 3 g; Iron 2 mg; Sodium 290 mg; Calcium 92 mg; Folate 77 mcg; Beta-Carotene 1,996 mcg; Potassium 578 mg

Ginger Egg Fried Rice

Grace Young is the author of the award-winning cookbook *The Wisdom of the Chinese Kitchen*. It seemed fitting that I should turn to her for a recipe that has the healing powers of traditional Chinese ingredients. Here's the fascinating history of this dish.

This light, vegetarian fried rice dish is recommended during and after pregnancy in China. In particular, the dish's ginger is good for combating nausea, and according to ancient Chinese wisdom, after their babies are born, some women lose their appetite from having a "*cold* stomach," and the ginger helps warm the system. Eggs are regarded as the perfect yin yang food, and rice, especially in southern Chinese dishes, is considered to be a harmonizing food that's wonderful for all stages of life.

If not using a carbon-steel wok, Grace recommends a 12-inch stainless-steel skillet rather than a nonstick pan.

Note: The ginger should be shredded, not grated. Grating it makes the ginger too watery, and it will spatter in the pan. If you want a bit more protein, add 2 more eggs.

Prep: 8 minutes

Cook: 5 minutes

Makes 4 1-cup servings

Momma Must-Have: A feel-good food for your belly that cooks in just 5 minutes, plus it offers 4 g fiber!

2 tablespoons peanut or vegetable oil

2 tablespoons finely shredded ginger

4 cups cooked white or brown rice, cold

1 egg, beaten

½ cup chopped scallions

1 tablespoon reduced sodium soy sauce

¼ teaspoon salt

⅛ teaspoon ground white pepper

½ teaspoon Asian sesame oil

1. Heat a 14-inch flat-bottomed wok or large skillet over high heat until a bead of water vaporizes within 1 to 2 seconds of contact. Swirl in 1 tablespoon of the peanut oil, add the ginger, and stir-fry for 10 seconds. Add the rice and stir-fry for 3 minutes, separating the rice with a spatula.

2. Make a well in the rice, exposing the bottom of the wok. Add the remaining 1 tablespoon oil and the beaten egg. Immediately, stir-fry for 1 minute, incorporating the egg throughout the rice, or until egg is flecked throughout the mixture and just cooked through. Add the scallions, soy sauce, salt, and pepper, and stir fry for 1 minute until heated through and the soy sauce is evenly distributed. Stir in the sesame oil.

Calories 308; Fat 11 g (Sat 2 g, Mono 2 g, Poly 5 g); Cholesterol 54 mg; Protein 7 g; Carbohydrate 47 g; Sugars 1 g; Fiber 4 g; Iron 1 mg; Sodium 271 mg; Calcium 35 mg; Folate 16 mcg; Zinc 1 mg

SALTY/SAVORY

SALADS

Confetti Rice Salad

This healthy antioxidant- and fiber-packed salad has a great tanginess to it. If you shun oily dressing, take note: A 2004 study published in The American Journal of Clinical Nutrition found that you absorb more antioxidants (specifically carotenoids, which are important for healthy eyes) from salads when your salad is drizzled with full-fat dressing. In fact, no carotenoids were absorbed from salads with fat-free dressing. That's not to say you should go nuts with a bottle of creamy ranch, but adding heart-healthy extra-virgin olive oil to salads like this one is a smart way to boost nutrition. The carotenoids in this salad come from the cherry tomatoes.

Prep: 20 minutes

Makes 4 servings

Baby Bonus: This simple and delicious salad contains 20 percent of your daily calcium requirement to help form Baby's strong bones.

Momma Must-Have: Thanks to the garbanzo beans and brown rice, this salad packs in 8 g fiber to keep your digestion moving.

2 cups cooked brown rice (1 cup dry)

1 cup frozen peas, cooked

1 cup cherry tomatoes, halved

1 15-ounce can garbanzo beans, rinsed and drained

¼ cup Kalamata olives, sliced

⅓ cup cubed, pasteurized feta cheese

1½ tablespoons extra-virgin olive oil

1 tablespoon balsamic vinegar, preferably aged

Juice of ½ a large lemon

½ teaspoon salt

¼ teaspoon pepper

1 tablespoon chopped fresh mint (optional)

1. In a large mixing bowl, combine rice with peas, tomatoes, garbanzo beans, olives, and feta cheese. Set aside.

2. In a small bowl, whisk the oil and vinegar together. Add the lemon juice, salt, and pepper. Drizzle the dressing over the rice salad, and stir well with a spatula (or with clean hands—that's how I do it). Garnish with the fresh mint, if desired.

Calories 364; Fat 12 g (Sat 4 g, Mono 4 g, Poly 1 g); Cholesterol 11 mg; Protein 15 g; Carbohydrate 49 g; Sugars 3 g; Fiber 8 g; Iron 2 mg; Sodium 321 mg; Calcium 207 mg; Folate 10 mcg; Zinc 2 mcg

Roasted Beet, Pistachio, and Goat Cheese Salad with Basil Vinaigrette

If you don't have time to roast the beets (it's easy, but time consuming), pick some up at the salad bar; if you're really in a rush, go with canned. Just make sure to rinse them first (it helps remove the sugar and salt added during the canning process). If you make the beets yourself (definitely the best option for flavor and texture), you'll want to wear an apron, and maybe even plastic gloves to protect your clothes. Turn this into a main course by adding grilled chicken, fish, or tofu on top.

Prep: 10 minutes

Cook: 65 minutes

Makes 4 servings

Baby Bonus: Folate for Baby's healthy spine (20 percent of what you need for the day).

Momma Must-Have: Plenty of fiber to keep things moving, plus iron to boost your energy level.

Salad

1 pound fresh beets (preferably a mixture of yellow and red), trimmed

1 large cucumber, peeled and sliced

1 4-ounce package pasteurized goat cheese, crumbled

½ cup pistachios, salted and roasted

2 tablespoons chopped red onion

Vinaigrette

2 tablespoons extra-virgin olive oil

1 tablespoon sherry vinegar

4 basil leaves, chiffonade (sliced thinly)

¼ teaspoon salt

¼ teaspoon pepper

1. Preheat oven to 400°F.

2. Wrap beets tightly in foil, and place in a roasting pan (or on a baking sheet) in the center of the oven.

3. Roast for 60 to 90 minutes, or until tender when poked with a fork (smaller beets take less time to cook).

4. Remove from the oven and cool (this can be done up to 2 days ahead; beets should be kept tightly wrapped in the refrigerator).

In the meantime, whisk olive oil, sherry vinegar, basil, salt, and pepper together to make the vinaigrette. Set aside.

5. Once cooled, rub beets with a paper towel until skin slides off. Discard skin. Quarter beets and place in a large, stain-proof bowl.

6. Add cucumber slices, goat cheese, pistachios, and red onion. Drizzle vinaigrette over salad. Toss gently and serve.

Calories 290; Fat 20 g (Sat 6 g, Mono 10 g, Poly 3 g); Cholesterol 13 mg; Protein 11 g; Carbohydrate 19 g; Sugars 12 g; Fiber 4 g; Iron 2 mg; Sodium 362 mg; Calcium 87 mg; Folate 110 mcg

Spinach and Pear Salad with Pomegranate Dressing

If you've never cut open a pomegranate, you might be in for a messy surprise. The best way to get the seeds out without staining your clothes and counter is to cut the fruit in half, and then submerge it in a bowl of water. Then you can use your fingers to remove the white pith, releasing the juicy seeds. Once you've freed all the pomegranate seeds, pour the contents of the bowl into a colander and transfer the seeds to paper towels to dry. If you don't have white balsamic vinegar, you can use the regular kind.

Prep: 10 minutes

Makes 4 servings

Baby Bonus: This little salad has a lot of bang for the calories. The pomegranate juice and seeds provide a nice dose of antioxidants, the walnuts add brain-boosting omega-3s, and a ton of beta-carotene keeps Baby's skin and eyes growing well.

Momma Must-Have: When you don't feel like eating much, this dish helps you sneak in a lot of nutrients in a small package. You get fiber, calcium, and bloat-beating potassium.

1 medium clove garlic, minced

2 teaspoons olive oil

1 teaspoon white balsamic vinegar

2 tablespoons pomegranate juice

1 teaspoon honey

¼ teaspoon salt

¼ teaspoon freshly ground black pepper

5-ounce package baby spinach

1 medium pear (Anjou or Bartlett),
cored and cut into slices (¼-inch)

¼ cup chopped walnuts

2 tablespoons fresh pomegranate seeds

1 ounce Parmesan cheese, shaved

1. Whisk together the garlic, oil, vinegar, pomegranate juice, honey, salt, and pepper in a small bowl. Set aside.

2. Place the spinach in a large serving bowl. Add the pear slices and walnuts and toss gently. Drizzle the dressing over the salad and toss again.

3. Divide the salad among 4 servings bowls. Sprinkle the pomegranate seeds and the Parmesan evenly over each serving.

Calories 145; Fat 9 g (Sat 2 g, Mono 2 g, Poly 4 g, Omega-3 1 g); Cholesterol 5 mg; Protein 5 g; Carbohydrate 14 g; Sugars 9 g; Fiber 3 g; Iron 1 mg; Sodium 275 mg; Calcium 125 mg; Folate 79 mcg; Beta-Carotene 2,000 mcg; Potassium 305 mg

Mediterranean Barley Salad

I love the nutty flavor of barley and its great chewy texture. If you have the patience to use hulled whole-grain barley and can find it, go for it—it's got more fiber and nutrients than pearled barley, but it takes longer to cook. Still, pearled barley has more fiber than white rice, pasta, or even brown rice. Save time and use quick-cooking barley.

Prep: 10 minutes

Cook: 30 minutes

Makes 6 servings

Baby Bonus: Barley has 2 mg of iron per 1 cup serving, 1.2 mg of zinc, 25 mcg of folate, and the B vitamins niacin, riboflavin, and thiamin.

Momma Must-Have: You're getting a great source of both soluble and insoluble fiber from the barley.

1 cup uncooked pearled barley

2½ cups water

¼ cup chopped roasted red peppers

6 artichoke hearts, coarsely chopped

6 green olives, sliced, pitted

¼ cup pasteurized feta cheese, crumbled

2 cloves garlic, finely minced

2 tablespoons finely minced flat-leaf parsley

1 tablespoon olive oil

¼ teaspoon salt

⅛ teaspoon freshly ground black pepper

1. Add the barley and water to a 2-quart saucepan, and bring to a boil. Reduce heat, and simmer until barley is tender, about 30

minutes. Remove from heat, and drain any excess water. Transfer to a large bowl, and set aside to cool.

2. While the barley is cooking, in a medium bowl, combine the roasted red peppers, artichoke hearts, olives, feta cheese, garlic, and parsley. Set aside.

3. Once the barley has cooled, stir in the olive oil, salt, and pepper. Combine the barley with the vegetable mixture and serve.

Calories 176; Fat 5 g (Sat 1 g, Mono 2 g, Poly 0 g); Cholesterol 3 mg; Protein 5 g; Carbohydrate 29 g; Sugars 1 g; Fiber 7 g; Iron 1 mg; Sodium 205 mg; Calcium 38 mg; Folate 3 mcg

The Wedge

If you've ever been to an old-school steak house, you've seen a variation of this on the menu. It's basically a wedge of iceberg lettuce, usually doused with blue-cheese dressing. I hadn't tried one till I went to Joe's Stone Crab in South Beach. Usually, I stay away from watery, nutrient-poor iceberg, but sometimes on a hot day it's really the most refreshing option. No blue cheese for you right now, but this buttermilk-dill dressing is also a nice match for the crisp lettuce.

Prep: 15 minutes

Makes 4 servings

Momma Must-Have: Dig into this fun salad, since it has only 81 calories and provides 4 g fiber and more than 10 percent of your calcium needs for the day.

Dressing

½ cup low-fat buttermilk

½ cup plain fat-free yogurt

¼ teaspoon salt

¼ teaspoon freshly ground black pepper

2 teaspoons chopped fresh dill

1 large clove garlic

1 head iceberg lettuce

1 medium cucumber, peeled and sliced into rounds

1 cup thinly sliced radishes (breakfast radishes can be used whole)

1 cup sugar snap peas, trimmed

1. Combine the buttermilk, yogurt, salt, pepper, dill, and garlic in a blender or food processor. Transfer to a jar or pitcher and place in the refrigerator.

2. Remove the outer leaves of the lettuce, cut out the core, and slice the head into 4 wedges. Place a wedge on each of 4 plates. Arrange the cucumber, radishes, and snap peas around each wedge.

3. Drizzle each salad with ¼ of the dressing and serve.

Calories 81; Fat 1 g (Sat 0 g, Mono 0 g, Poly 0 g); Cholesterol 3 mg; Protein 5 g; Carbohydrate 14 g; Sugars 9 g; Fiber 4 g; Iron 1 mg; Sodium 222 mg; Calcium 141 mg; Folate 71 mcg; Beta-Carotene 597 mcg

Warm Fig Salad with Pecans

There's something about fresh figs that just gets me. Maybe it's because I remember my mother telling me stories about she and my father devouring them on their honeymoon in Italy, or maybe it's their rich, meaty, and voluptuous texture. Either way, they are something to behold, but they're only in season from mid-summer to early fall. This salad is delicious with fresh or dried figs.

Prep: 5 minutes

Cook: 10 minutes

Makes 4 servings

Momma Must-Have: Figs are total nutrition stars. Packed with calcium, fiber, and potassium, they're an indulgent way to stay healthy.

6 fresh or dried figs

2 tablespoons extra-virgin olive oil, divided

1½ tablespoons white-wine vinegar

1 shallot, minced

¼ teaspoon salt

¼ teaspoon freshly ground black pepper

8 cups organic salad greens

½ cup pecans

1. Preheat oven to 350°F.

2. In a small bowl, toss figs with ½ tablespoon olive oil. Place on a baking sheet and bake for 10 minutes. Remove from oven and cool.

3. While the figs are baking, whisk together the remaining olive oil, vinegar, shallot, salt, and pepper in a bowl.

4. Slice cooled figs in half lengthwise. Place salad greens in a large serving bowl, and add the dressing, figs, and pecans, and toss. Divide salad onto 4 plates and serve.

Calories 253; Fat 17.5g (Sat 2g, Mono 5g, Poly 1g); Cholesterol 0 mg; Protein 4 g; Carbohydrate 23 g; Sugars 9 g; Fiber 6 g; Iron 1 mg; Sodium 160 mg; Calcium 30 mg

Mustardy Green Bean and Cherry Tomato Salad

This dressing works equally well with boiled red potatoes and steamed asparagus.

Prep: 15 minutes

Cook: 10 minutes

Makes 6 servings

Baby Bonus: This salad has a good dose of folate and beta-carotene for Baby.

Momma Must-Have: This recipe is super-low cal, so it's great for those times when you're feeling like the Hindenburg.

1 pound green beans, trimmed

1 pint cherry tomatoes, halved (a combo of red and yellow is nice)

2 tablespoons Dijon mustard

2½ tablespoons extra-virgin olive oil

2 tablespoons sherry vinegar

¼ teaspoon sea salt or kosher salt

¼ teaspoon freshly ground black pepper

1. Bring a large pot of water to a boil. Meanwhile, place a colander in the sink with ice cubes.

2. Once the water boils, drop in the green beans. Allow to boil until the color of the beans brightens, about 2 minutes. Drain beans, and immediately place in the colander with ice, allowing cold water to run over the beans until they become cool to the touch. Drain.

3. Place the beans in a medium bowl along with the tomatoes. Set aside.

4. Whisk together the mustard, olive oil, sherry vinegar, salt, and

pepper. Drizzle over the vegetables and toss. Serve alongside chicken, fish, or pork.

Calories 86; Fat 6 g (Sat 1 g, Mono 4 g, Poly 1 g); Cholesterol 0 mg; Protein 2 g; Carbohydrate 8 g; Sugars 2 g; Fiber 3 g; Iron 1 mg; Sodium 178 mg; Calcium 30 mg; Folate 32 mcg, Beta-Carotene 475 mcg

SOUPS

Miso Pretty Soup

I always feel really healthy after a bowl of miso soup. Miso paste is made from fermented soybeans. It comes in various varieties, from white to red. Generally, the darker the color, the stronger the flavor. Miso is high in fiber and zinc.

Prep: 10 minutes

Cook: 10 minutes

Makes 4 servings (small ones, like what you'd get in a Japanese restaurant)

Momma Must-Have: This low-cal, low-fat soup is the perfect picker-upper when you're feeling a bit under the weather. The tofu nets you about 9 percent of your daily calcium.

5 cups water

1 cup cubed firm tofu

2 cups packed spinach leaves

¼ cup sliced scallions, white and light green parts only

1 cup sliced shiitake mushrooms

⅓ cup white miso (soy bean paste)

¼ teaspoon sea salt

1. Bring the water to a boil. Reduce to medium heat, and add the tofu, spinach, scallions, and mushrooms. Simmer for 10 minutes.

2. Turn heat off, and stir in miso until fully dissolved. Add the salt and serve.

Calories 101; Fat 2 g (Sat 0 g, Mono 0 g, Poly 0 g); Cholesterol 0 mg; Protein 9 g; Carbohydrate 11 g; Sugars 2 g; Fiber 1 g; Iron 1 mg; Sodium 552 mg; Calcium 89 mg; Folate 21 mcg; Beta-Carotene 399 mcg

Roasted Fall Vegetable Soup

If you have a hankering for this soup in the summer and can't find butternut squash or any other winter squash, substitute Yukon Gold potatoes. And if you absolutely can't stand kale (try it anyway…I think this soup will change your mind), you can substitute spinach or Swiss chard.

Prep: 15 minutes

Cook: 1 hour and 10 minutes

Makes 6 servings

Baby Bonus: This soup is antioxidant-packed! It meets your beta-carotene and vitamin C needs for the day, so your little one's new cells can develop and fight off free radicals at the same time.

Momma Must-Have: Make this hearty soup on Sunday, and you'll have healthy, fiber-packed meals until Wednesday.

2 tablespoons olive oil, divided

1 large sweet potato, peeled and diced into 1-inch pieces

1 small butternut squash, peeled, seeded,
and diced into 1-inch pieces

2 parsnips, peeled and sliced into rounds

¼ teaspoon salt

¼ teaspoon pepper

1 large onion, diced

1 large bunch kale, chopped (about 10 cups)

2 16-ounce cartons low sodium organic chicken or vegetable broth

2 sprigs fresh thyme, plus 2 teaspoons chopped thyme

1 dried bay leaf

1 15-ounce can black-eyed peas

1. Preheat the oven to 400°F.

2. Drizzle 1 tablespoon of the oil in the bottom of a 9x13-inch roasting pan. Place the sweet potato, squash, and parsnips in the pan. Add the salt and pepper, and toss until well mixed. Put the pan in the oven, and bake for 40 minutes, or until vegetables are fork-tender.

3. Meanwhile, add the remaining tablespoon of oil to a large stock pot. Heat over medium-high heat for a minute, and then add the onion. Reduce heat to medium-low, and cook until onions are lightly golden, about 3 to 5 minutes.

4. Add the chopped kale to the pot, and cook for 2 minutes, until wilted. Add the broth to the pot, along with the thyme and bay leaf. Increase heat to medium, cover and bring to a boil. Reduce heat to low and simmer, covered, for 20 minutes.

5. Add the black-eyed peas to the pot, and simmer for an additional 5 minutes. Add additional salt and pepper to taste, if necessary. Remove bay leaf. Serve in large bowls with crusty whole-grain bread.

Calories 182; Fat 4.5 g (Sat 1 g, Mono 3 g, Poly 1 g, Omega-3 170 mg); Cholesterol 2 mg; Protein 7 g; Carbohydrate 33 g; Sugars 5 g; Fiber 7 g; Iron 3 mg; Sodium 632 mg; Calcium 192 mg; Vitamin C 126 mg; Folate 62 mcg; Beta-Carotene 10,908 mcg; Potassium 914 mg; Niacin 2 mg

Sweetie-Pie Sweet Potato Soup

This delicious, smooth, soothing soup is such a treat, it's hard to believe it's so good for you. But it's packed with 100 percent of your daily vitamin A needs (in the form of beta-carotene). If you're serving this to guests, or just feeling a bit decadent, add a dollop of crème fraîche and a sprinkling of toasted walnuts. Hang onto this recipe for when Junior is ready for pureed foods—he can eat it, too, minus the salt and pepper.

Prep: 20 minutes

Cook: 27 minutes

Makes 6 servings

Baby Bonus: Tons of beta-carotene ensures that Baby's vision gets a healthy start.

Momma Must-Have: The rich potassium content of this soup helps balance your sodium level and beat the bloat. The 7 g fiber don't hurt in that department either.

2 tablespoons unsalted butter or olive oil

1 medium onion, chopped

1 large clove garlic, sliced

2 pounds sweet potatoes, peeled and cut into pieces (1-inch)

4 cups organic chicken broth

3 whole cloves

1 cinnamon stick

¼ teaspoon ground nutmeg

1 cup organic 1% milk

¼ teaspoon salt

¼ teaspoon freshly ground black pepper

2 tablespoons crème fraîche, for serving (optional)

2 tablespoons chopped, toasted walnuts, for garnish (optional)

1. Heat the butter or olive oil in a large stock pot.

2. Add the onion and cook for 3 to 5 minutes over medium heat, until onion is translucent. Add the garlic, and cook for an additional 2 minutes.

3. Add the sweet potatoes, broth, and spices, and bring to a boil. Reduce the heat and simmer until the sweet potatoes are tender, about 20 minutes.

4. Using a slotted spoon, remove the cloves and cinnamon stick from the mixture. Carefully transfer the hot potato mixture to a blender in 3 batches. **Caution**: Do not fill the blender all the way to the top, as the steam may cause the lid to pop off. Blend until creamy and transfer to a bowl. Once the entire mixture is puréed, return it to the stock pot, and heat over medium-low.

5. Add the milk, salt, and pepper, and stir to combine. Ladle into bowls, and serve with a teaspoon each of crème fraîche and toasted walnuts, if desired. Leftovers can be refrigerated for up to three days.

Calories 212; Fat 5 g (Sat 3 g, Mono 0 g, Poly 0 g); Cholesterol 16 mg; Protein 5 g; Carbohydrate 38 g; Sugars 14 g; Fiber 7 g; Iron 2 mg; Sodium 555 mg; Calcium 136 mg; Folate 10 mcg; Beta-Carotene 17,402 mcg

PASTAS

Brocco Mac and Cheese

The ultimate comfort food grows up a little in this healthy version. It's still rich and cheesy, but it also gets extra calcium from the dried milk powder and the broccoli. The top gets nice and crunchy from the breadcrumbs.

Prep: 5 minutes

Cook: 33 minutes

Makes 6 servings

Baby Bonus: More than 30 percent of your daily calcium needs— for Baby's growing bones—wrapped up in cheesy goodness.

Momma Must-Have: You get to indulge your comfort food craving without feeling the least bit guilty.

2 cups organic 1% milk

1 tablespoon nonfat dried milk powder

1 tablespoon unsalted butter

2 tablespoons all-purpose flour

6 ounces organic shredded cheddar cheese

¼ teaspoon salt

¼ teaspoon freshly ground black pepper

1 10-ounce package frozen chopped broccoli, thawed

8 ounces whole-wheat macaroni, cooked

¼ cup dry breadcrumbs

1 tablespoon grated Parmesan cheese

1. Preheat oven to 350°F. Spray an 11x7-inch baking dish with cooking spray. Set aside.

2. Combine the milk with the milk powder in a measuring cup or small bowl. Set aside.

3. Melt the butter in a large saucepan over medium heat. Whisk in the flour. Cook, stirring constantly for two minutes.

4. Add the milk gradually, whisking after each addition. Cook for

a total of 5 minutes until mixture thickens, whisking constantly. Remove from heat.

5. Add the cheddar cheese, salt, and pepper to the warm milk mixture. Stir with a wooden spoon until the cheese melts, about a minute. Stir in the broccoli and cooked macaroni. Transfer mixture to the prepared baking dish, sprinkle the breadcrumbs and Parmesan on top, and put in the oven.

6. Bake for 25 to 30 minutes, until golden on top. Let sit for 5 minutes before digging in.

Calories 276; Fat 13 g (Sat 7 g, Mono 0 g, Poly 0 g); Cholesterol 41 mg; Protein 16 g; Carbohydrate 28 g; Sugars 6 g; Fiber 3 g; Iron 1 mg; Sodium 383 mg; Calcium 360 mg; Folate 37 mcg; Beta-Carotene 290 mcg

Farfalle with Edamame and Pecorino

Simple yet delicious, this protein-rich pasta dish is a weeknight star. Use a vegetable peeler to shave the pecorino cheese: it works like a charm.

Prep: 5 minutes

Cook: 20 minutes

Makes 6 servings

Baby Bonus: Baby gets almost 30 percent of the daily requirement for folate, which helps him build a healthy spine.

Momma Must-Have: Thanks to the edamame, you get 6 g fiber, 10 percent of your daily calcium, and a third of your protein needs for the day.

16-ounce package dried farfalle pasta

½ cup organic chicken broth

2½ cups frozen shelled edamame

2 teaspoons extra-virgin olive oil

¼ teaspoon salt

¼ teaspoon freshly ground black pepper

⅓ cup shaved pecorino cheese

1. Bring a large pot of water to boil on the stove.

2. In a large skillet, add the broth and edamame. Bring to a simmer over medium-high heat. Simmer for 10 minutes, then turn to low. The broth should reduce by half.

3. When the water boils, add the farfalle and cook according to the package directions. Drain.

4. Transfer the pasta to a large serving dish, and add in the edamame and any remaining broth. Stir in the olive oil, salt, and pepper. Divide the pasta among six serving bowls, and top with the shaved pecorino.

Calories 397; Fat 7 g (Sat 2 g, Mono 1 g, Poly 0 g); Cholesterol 5 mg; Protein 21 g; Carbohydrate 62 g; Sugars 6 g; Fiber 6 g; Iron 5 mg; Sodium 257 mg; Calcium 108 mg; Folate 162 mcg; Zinc 1 mg

VEGETABLE SIDES

Roasted Spring Asparagus

Once roasted, asparagus become even sweeter. This dish is fantastic with lamb or salmon, or just on top of a bed of greens. They're also quite good eaten with your fingers—you can feed them to your husband. I like making extra hard-boiled eggs with this recipe. They're a great quick protein source.

Prep: 8 minutes

Cook: 30 minutes

Makes 6 to 8 servings

Baby Bonus: This recipe gives you more than half your daily folate requirement! That'll keep Baby's spinal cord and neural tubes growing well.

4 eggs (preferably omega-3 enhanced)

24 thin asparagus spears, woody ends trimmed (about 2 pounds)

1 tablespoon olive oil

Salt (to taste)

Freshly ground black pepper (to taste)

2 teaspoons truffle oil (or a good extra-virgin olive oil)

1. Preheat oven to 425°F.

2. Put a medium pot of water on the stove. Gently add the eggs to the pan and bring to a boil.

3. Meanwhile, drizzle olive oil in a roasting pan or baking sheet.

4. Lay asparagus evenly in pan. Season with salt and pepper. Put in the oven for 20 minutes or until the stalks are *al dente*.

5. Allow the eggs to sit in the boiling water for 10 minutes, then turn the heat off. Drain and let cool.

6. Chop 2 of the eggs and set aside. Refrigerate the other 2, and use them later in a salad, or just as a snack.

7. Place the asparagus on a large platter, drizzle with a little truffle oil (or good extra-virgin olive oil), and sprinkle the chopped eggs on top. Serve warm or at room temperature.

Calories 103; Fat 6 g (Sat 1 g, Mono 3 g, Poly 1 g, Omega-3 100 mcg); Cholesterol 71 mg; Protein 7 g; Carbohydrate 9 g; Sugars 3 g; Fiber 4 g; Iron 2 mg; Sodium 53 mg; Calcium 57 mg; Folate 322 mcg

Smashed Edamame and Potatoes with Miso

Mark Bittman has visited most American households—maybe not literally, but virtually through his many cookbooks, including *How to Cook Everything*. His straightforward, no-nonsense style has always been a favorite of mine, and I've been lucky enough to get to know

Mark personally. He shared this easy, nutritious recipe with me, and now I have the pleasure of sharing it with you.

Prep: 10 minutes

Cook: 25 minutes

Makes 4 to 6 servings

Momma Must-Have: This recipe is the perfect way to sneak in some extra nutrition during those times when your stomach can't handle much more than mashed potatoes. You'll get a little protein, fiber, iron, and potassium in an easy-to-handle dish.

2 medium potatoes, peeled and cubed

2 cups edamame, fresh or frozen

2 to 3 tablespoons miso, mixed
with ¼ cup hot water

Salt (to taste)

Freshly ground black pepper (to taste)

Chopped scallion, for garnish (optional)

1. Boil the potatoes in water to cover until soft, about 20 minutes.

2. Meanwhile, in another pot, bring about 1 quart water to a boil; add the edamame and cook for 5 to 7 minutes. Drain the edamame, reserving the cooking liquid, and transfer to a blender

or food processor. Pulse until roughly chopped (leave some of the beans whole). If using a blender, add a few tablespoons of the reserved liquid.

3. Drain the potatoes when done, reserving some of the cooking liquid. In a large bowl, combine the potatoes, edamame, and miso. Smash the mixture with a masher or wooden spoon (it should be fairly chunky). Add a little of the reserved cooking liquid if the mixture is too dry. Taste and adjust the seasoning, adding salt and pepper or more miso as needed. Garnish with scallion, if desired, and serve.

Reprinted from *How to Cook Everything* by Mark Bittman with permission from John Wiley and Sons, Inc.

Calories 98; Fat 2 g (Sat 0 g, Mono 0 g, Poly 0 g); Cholesterol 0 mg; Protein 7 g; Carbohydrate 13 g; Sugars 2 g; Fiber 3 g; Iron 2 mg; Sodium 190 mg; Calcium 24 mg; Folate 4 mcg; Potassium 139 mg

Mean Greens and Beans

This is one of those vegetarian recipes that has it all: protein, fiber, calcium, vitamin C, iron, and potassium. It's a great side dish for beef, chicken, or tofu, or just toss it with penne.

Prep: 10 minutes

Cook: 12 minutes

Makes 4 servings

Baby Bonus: Calcium and beta-carotene to keep Baby's bones and skin growing nicely. This recipe also contains almost 20 percent of your zinc requirement, which is important for regulating gene expression.

Momma Must-Have: You get 3 mg iron to stay strong, 6 g fiber to fight constipation, and 100 percent of your vitamin C for the day—all in only 149 calories!

1 tablespoon olive oil

1 clove garlic, minced

¼ teaspoon crushed red pepper

10 ounces (1 big bunch) kale, chopped

1 15-ounce can cannellini beans, rinsed and drained

½ cup organic chicken broth

¼ teaspoon salt

¼ teaspoon freshly ground black pepper

1. Heat the olive oil over medium-high heat in a large sauté pan. Add the garlic and red pepper, and cook until garlic is golden and fragrant, about 3 minutes.

2. Add the kale to the pan, and cook until wilted, about 3 to 4 minutes. Transfer kale to a colander to drain.

3. Add the beans and broth to the pan, and heat over medium-high heat. Simmer for 5 minutes, and return the kale to the pan. Add the salt and pepper and serve.

Calories 149; Fat 5 g (Sat 1 g, Mono 3.5 g, Poly 1 g); Cholesterol 0 mg; Protein 7 g; Carbohydrate 21 g; Sugars 1 g; Fiber 6 g; Iron 3 mg; Sodium 209 mg; Calcium 130 mg; Folate 21 mcg; Vitamin C 85 mg; Beta-Carotene 6,564 mcg; Potassium 527 mg; Zinc 2 mg

Grilled Vegetables in the Style of Santa Margherita

My friend Steven Raichlen is known as the Grilling Guru. His instructive books on grilling have sold millions and have gotten a lot of Americans fired up about grilling—including me. This is a pretty basic but delicious recipe for grilled veggies. It might seem like a ton of food, but once they are grilled, vegetables will keep for as long as three days. You can use the leftovers to make a salad or grilled veggie sandwiches, or chop and toss them with pasta.

Prep: 35 minutes

Cook: 20 minutes

Makes 6 servings

Baby Bonus: This recipe contains more than 200 percent of your daily vitamin C needs, helping Baby's skin form beautifully. A healthy amount of folate and potassium make this a nutritional winner too.

Basil oil:

¼ cup extra-virgin olive oil

2 to 4 fresh basil leaves, roughly chopped

1 large clove garlic, roughly chopped

1 teaspoon fresh lemon juice

Vegetables:

4 to 5 miniature or 2 regular red bell peppers,
seeded and halved

4 to 5 miniature or 2 regular orange bell peppers,
seeded and halved

4 to 5 miniature or 2 regular yellow bell peppers,
seeded and halved

1 head Belgian endive, cut lengthwise into quarters,
stem end attached

1 small head radicchio or Treviso (see note),
cut lengthwise into quarters, stem end attached

½ pound fresh cremini or button mushrooms,
stemmed, caps wiped clean with dampened paper towels

2 small zucchini, halved lengthwise

1 fennel bulb, cut into slices (⅜-inch), fronds removed

½ pound medium-thick asparagus, fibrous ends removed

4 small plum tomatoes

Coarse kosher or sea salt (to taste)

Freshly ground black pepper (to taste)

Lemon wedges, for serving

Balsamic vinegar (optional)

1. Make the basil oil: In a blender or food processor, combine the olive oil, basil, garlic, and lemon juice. Let sit for 30 minutes for flavors to develop.

2. Preheat the grill to medium-high. Preheat a vegetable grate (if using) for 5 minutes. Lightly brush the bell pepper pieces with the basil oil, season with the salt and pepper, and arrange on the hot grate. Grill until lightly charred on both sides, leaving the skins intact, 3 to 4 minutes per side. Transfer to a platter. Oil, season, and grill the endive, radicchio, mushrooms, zucchini, fennel, asparagus, and tomatoes the same way. Each vegetable should be nicely charred on the outside and soft and tender inside; depending on the vegetable, this will take 3 to 6 minutes per side. Brush all the vegetables lightly with the basil oil, and season with salt and pepper as they cook.

3. Arrange the grilled vegetables attractively on a platter. Drizzle the remaining oil on top of the hot vegetables, and let them cool.

4. Just before serving, you might want to season them again with salt and pepper. (Taste them to make sure.) Serve lemon wedges

on the side for squeezing over the vegetables. Alternatively, drizzle a bit of balsamic vinegar over the vegetables.

Note: Treviso is a colorful (burgundy) version of endive; look for it in specialty produce markets or order it from www.melissas.com.

Excerpted from *The Barbecue Bible* Copyright 1998, 2008 by Steven Raichlen. Used by permission of Workman Publishing Co., Inc., New York. All rights reserved.

Calories 163; Fat 10 g (Sat 1 g, Mono 7 g, Poly 1 g); Cholesterol 0 mg; Protein 4 g; Carbohydrate 17 g; Sugars 7 g; Fiber 6 g; Iron 1 mg; Sodium 227 mg; Calcium 61 mg; Vitamin C 189 mg; Folate 74 mcg; Beta-Carotene 1,027 mcg; Potassium 917 mg

OTHER TASTY THINGS

All-Purpose Veggie Dip

Trying to choke down some fresh veggies because you know you should? It can be tough work sometimes. Make it easier without blowing a ton of calories with this easy five-minute dip.

Prep: 5 minutes

Makes 5 servings

Momma Must-Have: If it gets you to eat some fresh veggies when you're not feeling up to it, this recipe is worth its weight in gold. It's low-cal and provides a decent amount of calcium.

¼ cup reduced-fat cream cheese with chives

½ cup reduced-fat cottage cheese

¼ cup reduced-fat pasteurized feta cheese

¼ cup roughly chopped flat-leaf parsley (optional)

1 tablespoon organic 1% milk

1. (Yes—only one step!) In a small food processor, add the cream cheese, cottage cheese, feta, and parsley, if using. Pulse until fully

combined. Then add the milk and pulse again. Serve with veggies or pretzels. Can be stored in an airtight container in the fridge for 3 days; stir before using.

Calories 49; Fat 3 g (Sat 2 g, Mono 0 g, Poly 0 g); Cholesterol 11 mg; Protein 4 g; Carbohydrate 3 g; Sugars 2 g; Fiber 0 g; Iron 0 mg; Sodium 209 mg; Calcium 70 mg

Pesto Pizza Pie

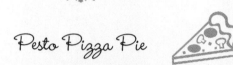

I don't know about you, but pizza is usually a once-in-a-while food for me. But during my first trimester, when I was in my salty-carb phase, I indulged in it quite frequently. In fact, I remember devouring a personal pizza on a flight back from Chicago, while my seatmate watched with more than a little amusement. This pizza has lots of great flavor without overloading you with sodium. Try it with any ingredients you like.

Prep: 5 minutes

Cook: 8 minutes

Makes 4 2-slice servings

Baby Bonus: This is a great bone-builder for Baby. You get more than 30 percent of your calcium requirement for the day.

1 10-ounce whole-wheat ready-made pizza crust

¼ cup prepared pesto

6 ounces fresh organic pasteurized mozzarella cheese, sliced into rounds

¼ cup pitted, halved kalamata olives

⅓ cup sun-dried tomatoes (not in oil), sulfur dioxide–free

⅓ cup marinated artichoke hearts, quartered

1. Preheat oven according to the directions on the pizza crust package.

2. Spread the pesto over the top of the crust, then top with mozzarella cheese, olives, sun-dried tomatoes, and artichoke hearts.

3. Bake for 8 to 10 minutes, until cheese is melted. Let sit for 5 minutes. Cut into 8 equal pieces and serve.

Calories 331; Fat 19 g (Sat 7 g, Mono 1 g, Poly 0 g); Cholesterol 28 mg; Protein 17 g; Carbohydrate 29 g; Sugars 3 g; Fiber 5 g; Iron 1 mg; Sodium 656 mg; Calcium 353 mg; Folate 3 mcg

Matzah Brei

This is a traditional Passover recipe, but it's not served at a seder. It's more of a homey, breakfast dish. It's not pretty, but it's super-easy and really hits the spot. My mom made it for me when I was a kid, and I've always loved it. If you can't find matzah (or just don't like it), you can also use whole-wheat crackers.

Prep: 5 minutes

Cook: 5 minutes

Makes 1 serving (can easily be doubled or tripled)

Baby Bonus: This recipe contains almost a third of your daily protein needs to keep Baby growing strong—plus 10 percent of your all-important iron and calcium needs, too.

Momma Must-Have: Vitamin B_{12} is vital for forming new blood cells (remember, your blood volume is increasing by 50 percent!) and for pretty much all of your body functions, which are working overtime right now.

1 teaspoon sugar

$1/8$–$1/4$ teaspoon ground cinnamon

2 eggs (preferably omega-3 enhanced)

3 tablespoons organic 2% or calcium-fortified soy milk

Pinch salt

1 teaspoon unsalted butter

½ sheet whole-wheat matzah (or 10 crackers),
broken into pieces

1. In a small bowl, combine the sugar and cinnamon and set aside (if you think you'll be making this often, mix up a bunch of cinnamon sugar and put it in a shaker or jar).

2. Crack the eggs into a small bowl and whisk them together. Add the milk and salt and mix well.

3. Melt the butter in a medium pan over medium-high heat. Add the egg mixture and broken matzah to pan.

4. Cook as you would scrambled eggs, pushing the mixture around the pan with a heatproof spatula. Cook until the eggs no longer look wet, about 3 to 4 minutes. For crispier edges, turn off the heat, but leave in the pan for a few minutes longer.

5. Transfer to a plate, top with cinnamon-sugar, and enjoy.

Calories 239; Fat 11 g (Sat 4 g, Mono 4 g, Poly 1 g, Omega-3 300 mg); Cholesterol 427 mg; Protein 17 g; Carbohydrate 20 g; Sugars 8 g; Fiber 2 g; Iron 3 mg; Sodium 159 mg; Calcium 114 mg; Folate 49 mcg; Vitamin B_{12} 1.5 mcg

SPICY

MAIN DISHES

Alisa's Taco Salad with Yogurty Salsa

During the early stage of my friend Alisa's pregnancy, she had a serious craving for Taco Bell. But instead of taking the easy route and heading for the drive-through, she drove home and made a taco salad, which is the inspiration behind this recipe. Depending on whether you're dealing with heartburn, you can kick up the level of spice to suit your taste.

Prep: 10 minutes

Cook: 8 minutes

Makes 4 servings

Baby Bonus: Wow, this salad is packed with good stuff! Baby gets 30 mg protein (half of what you need for the day) for growth, plus a ton of iron and B_{12} for healthy red blood cells.

Momma Must-Have: You get 45 percent of the zinc you need for the day to help ward off pesky colds, and 10 percent of your daily calcium needs to keep your bones strong. Plus, 10 g fiber knocks out about a third of your requirement for the day.

1 pound lean ground bison or sirloin

½ teaspoon ground cayenne pepper

½ teaspoon ground cumin

½ cup plus 3 tablespoons salsa, divided (hotness of your choice)

1 15-ounce can black beans, rinsed and drained

2 tablespoons light sour cream

8 cups chopped romaine (about 1 head)

1 avocado, diced

1 medium tomato, chopped

2 tablespoons fresh cilantro, for garnish

1. Remove the meat from the fridge ten minutes before cooking and allow to come to room temperature.

2. Add meat to a large pan, and cook over medium heat, breaking up with a spatula. Add the cayenne and cumin, and cook 6 to 7 minutes, or until there is no pink tint left to the meat. Remove from the heat, and drain off the juices (it might be good to ask for help with this if you have a large, heavy pan).

3. Stir ½ cup salsa and the beans into the meat and return to medium heat. Cook about 2 minutes, or until heated through. Season to taste with additional cayenne, salt, and pepper, if desired.

4. Meanwhile, in a small bowl, whisk together the 3 tablespoons salsa and the sour cream. Set aside.

5. Divide the lettuce equally into serving bowls. Top with the meat mixture, tomato, and avocado. Drizzle with the dressing, garnish with cilantro, and serve.

Calories 340; Fat 13 g (Sat 4 g, Mono 7 g, Poly 2 g); Cholesterol 63 mg; Protein 30 g; Carbohydrate 28 g; Sugars 9 g; Fiber 10 g; Iron 5 mg; Sodium 384 mg; Calcium 122 mg; Folate 196 mcg; Beta-Carotene 4,072 mcg; Vitamin B_{12} 2.4 mcg; Potassium 564 mg; Zinc 5 mg

Huevos Rancheros Wrap

I love the flavors of traditional huevos rancheros, but the restaurant-style ones are loaded with fat. This version uses Napa cabbage instead of iceberg for more nutrition and whole-grain wraps instead of tortillas.

Prep: 10 minutes

Cook: 10 minutes

Makes 4 servings

Baby Bonus: The eggs in this delicious wrap provide about 30 percent of your daily choline for Baby's healthy brain development, plus 21 g protein and 4 mg iron.

Momma Must-Have: You get to indulge your spicy craving, while also getting more than 20 percent of the calcium and fiber you need for the day.

1 15-ounce can no-salt-added black beans, rinsed

4 eggs (preferably omega-3-enhanced)

¼ teaspoon salt

¼ teaspoon freshly ground black pepper

1 teaspoon olive oil

1 lime

1 avocado, peeled, seeded, and diced

1 cup salsa

4 10-inch whole-wheat wraps

½ cup organic Mexican-style shredded cheese

1 cup chopped Napa cabbage

1 vine-ripened tomato, diced

2 tablespoons chopped fresh cilantro (optional)

1. In a small pan, warm the beans over low heat, mashing lightly with a spatula. Keep the beans over low heat.

2. Whisk the eggs together, and add the salt and pepper. In a separate frying pan, heat the olive oil over medium heat. Add the eggs and lower the heat to medium-low. Move eggs around the pan with a heatproof spatula until scrambled, about 4 minutes.

3. Cut the lime in half. Squeeze one half over the chopped avocado. Cut the other half into wedges for serving; set aside.

4. In a heatproof container, microwave the salsa for about 40 seconds.

5. Place the wraps—one at a time—on a plain paper towel, and microwave for 30 seconds.

6. Place the wrap on a large plate, and in the center, place ¼ of the beans, eggs, cheese, salsa, and remaining toppings. Fold in ends of wrap, and begin rolling in from one end. Serve with a wedge of lime.

Calories 443; Fat 18 g (Sat 4 g, Mono 5 g, Poly 1 g, Omega-3 150 mg); Cholesterol 225 mg; Protein 21 g; Carbohydrate 50 g; Sugars 9 g; Fiber 11 g; Iron 4 mg; Sodium 776 mg; Calcium 228 mg; Vitamin C 29 mg; Folate 47 mcg; Potassium 353 mg

Not-Too-Spicy Thai Chicken Curry

When you get a craving for a spicy, creamy Thai curry, try this one before dialing for take-out. Most restaurant versions are loaded with extra oil and a ton of sodium. This version is much healthier, plus it comes together in less time than it would take for the delivery guy to show up.

Prep: 10 minutes

Cook: 12 minutes

Makes 4 servings

Baby Bonus: With a little over half the protein you need for the day, Baby gets a great burst for his growing body.

Momma Must-Have: You'll get 10 percent of the potassium and iron you need for the day, plus 4 g fiber.

1 13.5-ounce can light coconut milk

1¼ teaspoons green Thai curry paste

1 cup sliced (¼-inch) yellow or orange bell pepper

1 cup fresh or frozen broccoli florets

1 medium onion, chopped

1 tablespoon chopped fresh ginger

1 pound chicken breasts or tenders, cut into 2-inch pieces

1 tablespoon packed brown sugar

1½ teaspoons fish sauce

1 14.5-ounce can no-salt-added diced tomatoes, drained

1 tablespoon fresh lime juice

2 cups microwavable brown rice

1. Combine ½ cup of the coconut milk with the curry paste in a large skillet over medium-high heat. Bring to a boil, whisking continuously. Add the pepper, broccoli, onion, and ginger, and sauté for 5 minutes.

2. Add the chicken to the skillet, along with the remaining coconut milk, brown sugar, and fish sauce. Cook the chicken for about 3 minutes on each side, or until cooked through (a meat thermometer should register 165°F).

3. Stir in the tomatoes and lime juice, and heat through for another minute. In the meantime, microwave the rice for 90 seconds. Serve the curry over ½ cup rice.

Calories 358; Fat 8 g (Sat 5 g, Mono 1 g, Poly 1 g); Cholesterol 66 mg; Protein 32 g; Carbohydrate 38 g; Sugars 11 g; Fiber 4 g; Iron 3 mg; Sodium 501 mg; Calcium 49 mg; Folate 31 mcg; Potassium 528 mg; Zinc 2 mg

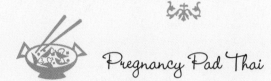

Pregnancy Pad Thai

I love the sweet-hot combination of this dish. Eat this on a day when you haven't had many other salty dishes, because the sodium is up there—1,000 mg. You can also omit the shrimp or tofu, or cut down on the fish sauce to reduce the sodium.

This recipe works especially well with one of those three-in-one pots that includes a colander and steam basket. You can get the shrimp already cleaned and deveined from the seafood counter at your grocery store.

Prep: 10 minutes

Cook: 25 minutes

Makes 6 servings

Baby Bonus: This isn't just pad Thai—it's pumped up specifically for pregnancy. It's got a ton more calcium (280 mg) and folic acid (111 mcg) from the bok choy, and lots of baby-building protein.

1 pound of rice noodles

1 bunch bok choy, white part only, cut into 1-inch pieces

3 tablespoons creamy peanut butter

2 tablespoons fish sauce

2 tablespoons low-sodium soy sauce

6 tablespoons organic chicken broth

2 teaspoons crushed red pepper

1 teaspoon sesame oil

2 tablespoons honey, such as orange blossom variety

1 tablespoon fresh lime juice (about 1 lime)

½ tablespoon vegetable oil

6 ounces marinated Asian-style tofu, cubed

¾ pound shrimp, shelled and deveined

1 egg, whisked

3 tablespoons fresh chopped cilantro

1 lime, quartered, for serving

1. Bring a large pot of water to a boil.

2. Add the noodles to the boiling water, and place the bok choy in the steamer basket above the noodles (or simply microwave for about 5 minutes). Cook noodles according to the package directions.

3. Meanwhile, whisk together the peanut butter, fish sauce, soy sauce, broth, chili flakes, sesame oil, honey, and lime juice in a medium bowl until combined. Set aside.

4. Remove the steamer basket (if using) with the bok choy, and set aside. Drain the pasta and run cold water over the noodles. Try to separate the noodles as much as possible (inevitably, some will stick together). Drain again and set aside.

5. Add the vegetable oil to a 12-inch skillet, and heat over medium-high heat.

6. Add the reserved bok choy to the skillet, and cook for 2 minutes. Add the tofu, and cook for another 2 minutes. Add the shrimp, and cook for about 1½ minutes per side until pink. Turn heat off, and transfer bok choy, tofu, and shrimp to a large bowl.

7. Using the same skillet, add reserved noodles to the pan and heat over low heat for about 2 minutes. Add the peanut butter mixture to the pan, and use tongs to turn the noodles, making sure sauce gets distributed evenly.

8. Add the reserved bok choy, tofu, and shrimp to the noodles, and heat over medium-high heat until warmed through.

9. Push mixture to the side of the pan and add the egg. Push the egg around in the pan until scrambled, about 45 seconds. Mix the cooked egg in with the rest of the ingredients.

10. Divide the noodle mixture among six bowls. Top with a sprinkling of cilantro, and place a lime wedge on the edge of the bowl.

Calories 483; Fat 11 g (Sat 2 g, Mono 3 g, Poly 3 g); Cholesterol 119 mg; Protein 19 g; Carbohydrate 78 g; Sugars 9 g; Fiber 3 g; Iron 6 mg; Sodium 1,000 mg; Calcium 280 mg; Folate 111 mcg; Vitamin C 65 mg; Beta-Carotene 3,906 mcg

SOUPS AND VEGGIES

Peasant-Style Gazpacho

If you're pregnant in the middle of the sweltering summer, this cold soup is a godsend. Not only is it light and refreshing, it'll also help keep you hydrated. Make it on a Sunday and enjoy it through Wednesday. The cubed bread (the drier it is, the better) will soak up a lot of the liquid, so you may want to add them with each serving instead of mixing into the entire batch.

Prep: 15 minutes

Chill: 1 hour

Makes 5 servings

Baby Bonus: Just a cup of this soup gives you all the vitamin C (85 mg) you need each day during pregnancy. Not only does it help you absorb the 3 mg iron in the gazpacho, it's also the glue that helps Baby's newly forming cells bind together.

Momma Must-Have: Gazpacho and other foods made with tomatoes, especially tomato sauce and juice, are packed with the antioxidant lycopene, which shows promise in helping first-time moms avoid preeclampsia. Just make sure you rely on food sources for lycopene, instead of supplements.

2 ounces (2 cups) day-old whole-grain bread, cubed

1 pound ripe tomatoes, preferably heirloom variety, diced

1 yellow or orange bell pepper, seeded and chopped

1 cucumber, peeled, seeded, and diced

¼ red onion, diced

1 tablespoon white or regular balsamic vinegar

1 teaspoon olive oil

¼ teaspoon chipotle chili powder

1 teaspoon salt

¼ teaspoon freshly ground black pepper

1 cup reduced-sodium tomato juice

½ pound cooked shrimp (optional)

2 tablespoons chopped cilantro, for garnish

1. Set the bread aside to dry out even more. Combine the tomatoes, bell pepper, cucumber, red onion, vinegar, olive oil, chili powder, salt, and black pepper in a large bowl.

2. Place ¾ of the gazpacho mixture into a blender. Add the tomato juice. Blend until soupy, but not entirely smooth. Pour gazpacho back into the bowl with the remaining unblended vegetables.

3. Chill for at least an hour before serving. Stir in the cubed bread and shrimp, if using. Garnish with cilantro and serve.

Fun things to add:

Cubed avocado

Diced hard-cooked egg

Asparagus tips

Calories 155; Fat 3 g (Sat 0.5 g, Mono 1 g, Poly 1 g); Cholesterol 111 mg; Protein 16 g; Carbohydrate 18 g; Sugars 9 g; Fiber 4 g; Iron 3 mg; Sodium 521 mg; Calcium 66 mg; Folate 53 mcg; Beta-Carotene 605 mcg; Vitamin C 91 mg

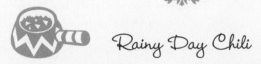

Rainy Day Chili

As its name suggests, this chili rocks on a cold, rainy day. Or any day you want a bit of spice and a hearty meal. I love this with a piece of corn bread and a sprinkle of Monterey Jack cheese on top. The cocoa powder adds an unexpected earthy-sweetness to the chili. Save time and use a rotisserie chicken—you'll get about 3 cups of meat from most of them.

Prep: 10 minutes

Cook: 40 minutes

Makes 8 servings

Baby Bonus: A bowl of this chili nets you ⅓ of the protein you need to keep baby growing strong each day.

Momma Must-Have: One serving gets you 20 percent closer to meeting your daily fiber quota. And 3 grams of iron keep you feeling strong.

1½ tablespoons olive oil

1 cup finely chopped onion

2 teaspoons ground cumin

½ teaspoon chipotle chili powder
(add more if you like it really spicy)

1 tablespoon unsweetened cocoa

2 15-ounce cans black beans, rinsed and drained

1 26-ounce container organic chicken broth

1 28-ounce can petite diced tomatoes, with juices

1½ cups frozen corn kernels

3 cups diced cooked chicken breast

1 yellow bell pepper, diced

½ cup chopped fresh cilantro

Salt and pepper (to taste)

1. Heat the oil over medium-high heat in a large stock pot. Add onion and sauté until soft, about 2 minutes. Add cumin, chili powder, cocoa, beans, and broth to pan. Cover, bring to a boil, reduce heat, and simmer for 20 minutes.

2. Using a ladle, remove 1½ cups of the bean mixture and transfer to a blender or food processor. If using a blender, remove the center part of the blender lid. Place the lid on the blender and cover the hole in the lid with a clean cloth. **Caution:** Carefully blend (a lot of steam will be coming off the mixture, so be sure to let some release) mixture until creamy. Return the mixture to the pot.

3. Add the tomatoes, corn kernels, chicken, and bell pepper, and cook over medium heat for 15 minutes. Add salt and pepper to taste. Stir in the cilantro and serve.

Calories 257; Fat 5 g (Sat 1 g, Mono 3 g, Poly 1 g); Cholesterol 47 mg; Protein 24 g; Carbohydrate 27 g; Sugars 9 g; Fiber 7 g; Iron 3 mg; Sodium 620 mg; Calcium 60 mg

Sesame-Ginger Green Beans

You've probably had something like this before at a Chinese restaurant, but no doubt they were loaded down with oil and sodium. This recipe is really easy to make, but the flavor is kick-ass if I do say so myself. It's excellent with salmon, chicken, or tofu.

Prep: 12 minutes

Cook: 10 minutes

Makes 4 servings

Momma Must-Have: This low-cal side dish has belly-soothing ginger, plus 4 g fiber to help you stay regular.

2 teaspoons olive oil

2 medium cloves garlic, minced

1 pound green beans, trimmed

3 teaspoons chopped fresh ginger

¼ teaspoon crushed red pepper

2 teaspoons toasted sesame oil

2 teaspoons maple syrup

1 teaspoon low-sodium soy sauce

1 tablespoon smooth peanut butter

1 tablespoon water

1. Heat the olive oil over medium-high heat in a large sauté pan.

2. Add the garlic and cook for 1 minute. Turn heat to low, and add beans. Cook for 5 minutes or until beans turn bright green.

3. While beans are cooking, in a small bowl, whisk together the ginger, pepper, sesame oil, maple syrup, soy sauce, peanut butter,

and water. Once beans are done cooking, add sauce to pan and toss well to coat beans. Cook for an additional 3 minutes. Serve with Ginger-Glazed Salmon (see recipe on page 201).

Calories 106; Fat 7 g (Sat 1 g, Mono 3 g, Poly 1 g); Cholesterol 0 mg; Protein 2.5 g; Carbohydrate 11 g; Sugars 5g; Fiber 4 g; Iron 1 mg; Sodium 48 mg; Calcium 60 mg; Folate 0 mcg; Potassium 298 mg

THIRST-QUENCHING

DAIRY

Nana-Berry Smoothie

This is much like the classic banana-mixed berry smoothie you love from the smoothie shop—without all the sugary extras they add in. And this mix is excellent for making frozen pops too.

Prep: 5 minutes

Makes 2 servings

Baby Bonus: Just one serving of this creamy, fruity drink gives Baby nearly 30 percent of the daily calcium requirement and 10 g protein.

1 large banana, sliced

1 cup frozen mixed berries

1 cup organic 1% milk or soy milk

6 ounces creamy-style low-fat organic raspberry yogurt

1 teaspoon honey (optional, if you need it sweeter)

1. Place ingredients in a blender, and blend until creamy and a pretty pink color. Pour half into a large glass, and save the rest for later, or share.

Calories 230; Fat 2 g (Sat 1.5 g, Mono 0.5 g, Poly 0 g); Cholesterol 13 mg; Protein 10 g; Carbohydrate 44 g; Sugars 33 g; Fiber 4 g; Iron 1 mg; Sodium 122 mg; Calcium 295 mg; Vitamin C 25 mg; Folate 14 mcg; Potassium 243 mg

Renée's Orange Creamsicle

When my friend Renée was pregnant with her second daughter, Riley, she began concocting OJ-based drinks in her blender. Her fave was a blend of orange juice and peanut butter. I've left that out of this recipe, but if you get a hankering for it, by all means, add a spoonful.

Prep: 5 minutes

Makes 2 servings

Baby Bonus: Baby gets almost 75 percent of the vitamin C requirement for the day, which helps her new cells form. If you use an omega-3 enhanced juice, you'll also get 50 mg omega-3.

1 cup orange juice

¼ cup organic 1% milk

1 tablespoon dry milk powder

½ cup organic low-fat vanilla yogurt

1. Place all ingredients in a blender, and blend until frothy. Pour into tall glasses and enjoy.

Calories 112; Fat 1 g (Sat 1 g, Mono 0 g, Poly 0 g); Cholesterol 6 mg; Protein 5 g; Carbohydrate 19 g; Sugars 17 g; Fiber 0 g; Iron 0 mg; Sodium 69 mg; Calcium 165 mg; Vitamin C 63 mg; Folate 38 mcg

NON-DAIRY

Gingery Watermelon Liquado

A liquado or licuado is basically a Mexican-style milkshake made with fresh fruit and either a splash of milk or water. They're sold by street vendors and are hugely popular. This version adds a kick of ginger beer, which makes this drink perfect for first-trimester belly woes.

Prep: 10 minutes

Makes 2 servings

Momma Must-Have: Look to this refreshing drink for lycopene, which may help prevent preeclampsia. The ginger beer also helps quell your queasy stomach.

2 cups diced, seedless watermelon

1 cup ice

2 tablespoons fresh lime juice

1 12-ounce bottle ginger beer
(such as Reed's Original Ginger Beer), chilled

1. Combine the melon, ice, and lime juice in a blender, and blend on high until liquefied.

2. Pour the mixture evenly into two tall glasses. Pour half of the ginger beer into each glass. Add more ice, if you like, and serve.

Calories 108; Fat 0 g (Sat 0 g, Mono 0 g, Poly 0 g); Cholesterol 0 mg; Protein 1 g; Carbohydrate 32 g; Sugars 30 g; Fiber 1g; Iron 0 mg; Sodium 10 mg; Calcium 12 mg; Folate 2 mcg; Beta-Carotene 304 mcg

Le Royale

As anyone who knows me can attest, my favorite drink of all time is the Kir Royale. It's really simple—just a little crème de cassis in the bottom of a champagne flute, topped off by the sparkly stuff. This was one thing I really hated to give up, so I created a drink that was the same shade of pink and equally as fabulous.

Prep: 3 minutes

Makes 1 serving

Momma Must-Have: This refreshingly light mocktail lets you feel like a sophisticated grown-up again. As you start prepping for baby talk, it's sometimes nice to steal away with one of these for a little alone time.

1 teaspoon black cherry juice concentrate (such as R.W. Knudsen)

3 ounces white grape juice, chilled

3 ounces sparkling water, chilled

1. Pour the black cherry juice concentrate into the bottom of a champagne flute or white wine glass. Add the grape juice and then the sparkling water. Put your feet up and daydream about wearing that amazing wrap dress that makes everyone's head turn.

Calories 48; Fat 0 g (Sat 0 g, Mono 0 g, Poly 0 g); Cholesterol 0 mg; Protein 0 g; Carbohydrate 12 g; Sugars 11 g; Fiber 0 g; Iron 0 mg; Sodium 1 mg; Calcium 13 mg; Folate 0 mcg

Love That Bump Lemonade

Many women told me that they couldn't get enough lemonade during their pregnancies, so I wanted to develop a lemonade recipe that was easy and not overly sugary. First, you've got to use fresh lemon juice (lime juice is super, too): the concentrate just doesn't cut it. Then you've got to sweeten it. This one's made with honey, which I find really delicious. If you prefer sugar, heat the same amount of natural sugar (or more if you've got a sweet tooth) with a cup of water on the stove until you get a syrup. This "simple syrup" then gets mixed with the lemon juice and water.

Prep: 10 minutes

Makes 8 8-ounce servings

Momma Must-Have: This tart beverage may just help nix your morning sickness—at least for a while.

8 ounces fresh lemon juice (about 5 lemons)

½ cup clover honey

64 ounces of cold water (8 cups)

Mint sprigs (optional)

1. After you've juiced all the lemons, set them aside. Place the honey in a heatproof container, and microwave it for 30 seconds. It should be nice and liquidy. If not, put it back in for another 10 seconds (don't do it for a full minute, or else it will get scalding hot).

2. Whisk the warm honey into the lemon juice. At this point, you can use the honey-lemon mixture as a concentrate, making a serving at a time and keeping the rest in a covered container in the fridge. Add ¼ cup of the concentrate to either cold water and ice for lemonade—sparkling water is a nice twist—or hot water for a soothing lemony beverage. Or you can add it to a big pitcher (filled up the rest of the way with the cold water), add a mint sprig (optional), and pour yourself a refreshing glass.

Calories 71; Fat 0 g (Sat 0 g, Mono 0 g, Poly 0 g); Cholesterol 0 mg; Protein 0 g; Carbohydrate 20 g; Sugars 17 g; Fiber 0 g; Iron 0 mg; Sodium 1 mg; Calcium 10 mg; Folate 7 mcg; Vitamin C 14 mg

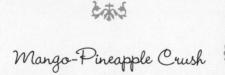

Mango-Pineapple Crush

Mango and pineapple are two of my favorite fruits. When you add the coconut sorbet, this becomes a tropical treat that might even be better than a piña colada (try it with a shot of rum post-baby). Can you say cabana boy?

Prep: 10 minutes (if you cut up your own pineapple)

Makes 2 servings

Momma Must-Have: You get a sweet, tropical indulgence for less than 200 calories, plus 40 percent of the vitamin C you need each day.

1 cup diced (1-inch) fresh pineapple

8-ounces mango juice (such as Looza or Ceres)

⅓ cup coconut sorbet

1 tablespoon shredded unsweetened coconut (optional)

1 cup ice

1. Combine all ingredients in a blender, and blend until smooth and creamy. Pour into a tall glass and pretend you're in Cabo.

Calories 167; Fat 3 g (Sat 2 g, Mono 0 g, Poly 0 g); Cholesterol 2 mg; Protein 1 g; Carbohydrate 36 g; Sugars 28 g; Fiber 1 g; Iron 1 mg; Sodium 10 mg; Calcium 37 mg; Vitamin C 34 mg; Folate 12 mcg

Belly Tip

The Best Way to Core a Pineapple

First, slice off both ends of the fruit. Now you should have a stable bottom base. Stand the pineapple on its bottom end. With one hand, stabilize the fruit. With the other, cut downward on all four sides, removing the thick outer skin. Cut away any remaining "eyes." You should have a solid rectangle of fruit. Now, all you need to do is cut the pineapple into quarters and slice away the stiff inner core. Then just cut the juicy fruit into chunks.

If that's too much work for today, buy the pineapple chunks from your grocery's refrigerated section.

Papaya Blue Lagoon

Ever since I sliced open my first papaya during a spring break trip to the Bahamas, I've been into this tropical fruit. But not everyone is, probably because it often comes with a funky smell. The flesh is sweet, with a satisfyingly rich texture.

Even if you're not a big fan of papaya, give this recipe a try. Not only is it packed with folic acid and antioxidants, but the blueberries really tone down the flavor of the papaya. Note: Do not eat unripe papaya! It contains latex, which can cause premature contractions.

Prep: 7 minutes

Makes 2 8-ounce servings

Baby Bonus: Antioxidant-rich blueberries help protect Baby's developing cells. Vitamin C and folate from the papaya also help ensure healthy growth.

Momma Must-Have: Fortified soy milk adds more than 10 percent of your calcium needs for the day.

1 cup ripe papaya, diced

¾ cup vanilla soy milk, chilled

¼ cup fresh or frozen blueberries

1 tablespoon fresh lime juice (optional)

1 teaspoon honey

1. Place all ingredients into a blender, and blend until smooth.

Calories 89; Fat 1 g (Sat 0 g, Mono 0 g, Poly 0 g); Cholesterol 0 mg; Protein 3 g; Carbohydrate 17 g; Sugars 11 g; Fiber 2 g; Iron 0.5 mg; Sodium 38 mg; Calcium 131 mg; Vitamin C 47 mg; Folate 37 mcg

Chapter Eighteen

The Milk Factory and Beyond

By now, you've brought home your little bundle and are dealing with an incredible mixture of joy, pain, fear, and utter exhaustion. Plus, a dairy farm just set up shop on your chest, and if you've decided to breast-feed, you can't slack off on your nutrition. In fact, most experts recommend that women who breast-feed consume 500 extra calories a day than what they ate before they were pregnant.[1] So, if you were eating 2,000 calories a day pre-pregnancy, you could go up to 2,500.

Try not to overthink everything you put in your mouth—Lord knows your sleep-deprived brain can only process so much right now. The important thing is that you stay well nourished and choose healthy, unprocessed foods as much as possible. Our bodies are pretty darned efficient, and we'll produce quality milk even if we're eating odd things at odd hours. The good news is that those (ahem) *reserves* you've accumulated during your pregnancy will now be put to good use.[2]

There are certain nutrients you need to keep in mind while you're breast-feeding. Keep eating lots of fresh fruits, veggies, and whole grains, and be sure to get plenty of lean protein. It's a good idea to continue taking your prenatal vitamin, just to cover all the bases, but check with your doctor to see if she agrees. Here are some of the biggies to keep in mind (requirements are per day):[3]

Vitamin C: 120 mg
Get it from fresh fruits, fruit juices, and vegetables.

Choline: 550 mg

Scramble up some eggs (or make the Huevos Rancheros Wrap on page 237) for a good supply.

Calcium: 1,000 mg

Keep on drinking your milk, eating your yogurt, and getting plenty of dark, leafy greens.

Zinc: 12 mg

Get a burst with fortified cereal and shrimp—not together, of course.

Potassium: 5,100 mg

It sounds like a ridiculous amount, but most foods contain at least some potassium. A banana has nearly 500 mg and a large baked potato has 1,600 mg.

Source: Institute of Medicine

Making breast milk requires a lot of water, so remember to stay hydrated. Your thirst should be a good indicator of when you need to drink more. And take a look in the toilet—if your pee is a nice light, lemonade color, you're well hydrated. If it's a dark amber color, get drinking. Remember that water-rich fruits and vegetables also help contribute to your water intake.

Laughter Is the Best Medicine

Get ready to add *There's Something About Mary* to your Netflix list. A study done in Osaka, Japan, showed that women who laughed prior to breast-feeding had higher levels of melatonin in their milk. It doesn't sound like a big deal until you consider that melatonin helps you relax, and people with eczema have reduced levels of melatonin. Indeed, when infants were fed the higher-melatonin milk, they were less reactive to dust mites and latex.[4] Even if you and your baby are eczema-free, just the idea that laughter can boost the relaxation quotient of your milk is reason enough to justify your weekly fill of *The Office.*

What about breast-feeding to help you lose weight? It's a hotly debated topic on blogs and among friends. For some women, it seems to work like a charm. I've seen friends and acquaintances drop weight really quickly just by breast-feeding, while other women who choose the breast struggle with their weight for a year or more. Breast-feeding burns as many as 500 calories a day, which should lead to one pound of weight loss per week.[5] But if you're taking in too many calories, it can still be tough to shed the pounds.

Exercise

You may have heard that you shouldn't exercise while you're breast-feeding because lactic acid created by your muscles can "sour" your milk. It sounds pretty rational, but a review of the studies on the subject found that any change in breast milk caused by exercise isn't likely to be a problem.[6] One study even showed that women who exercise actually produce more milk.[7]

Most new moms find that their pre-baby exercise schedule completely goes out the window once the little one arrives. But getting back to an exercise routine four to six weeks postpartum will not only help you get back in shape, but it'll also boost your mood and energy level, and give you some much-needed Me Time outside the house. Before you give birth, set up a schedule that allows you to get to the gym or meet a friend for a power walk (Baby can come, too) a few times a week. Knowing that you've got an "appointment" to exercise will make it easier to stick to it.

If you've had a C-section, you'll need time to heal. Talk to your doctor about when it's safe to go back to an exercise routine. If your baby arrives in the middle of winter, you'll need some incentive to exercise. Don't be shy about registering for a few exercise DVDs along with all the stuff for Baby.

Once you've been thrown into the world of onesies and Diaper Genies, it's hard to focus on weight loss. But I've got to tell you that sooner is better, as long as you feel up to it. Women who get back to their pre-pregnancy weight within six months have a lower risk of being overweight ten years down the road. And the women who lost the weight did it with a combination of diet and exercise, because diet alone didn't cut it.[8]

Conclusion

You're on the other side now, with a healthy baby cradled in your arms. And you're feeling great (well, beyond the breast pumping and the exhaustion) because you took really wonderful care of yourself for all nine months. Let me guess…with all the great food you've been eating, you didn't even miss the sushi and deli sandwiches. Keep up the great work, making sure you take the time to eat a mostly whole-food diet along with plenty of water. Gradually ease back into fitness to get your pre-pregnancy body back. The recipes in this book are also great postpartum, when you're rebuilding your nutrient stores and breast-feeding your new baby!

Hopefully, *Feed the Belly* helped you get through some tough days and cleared up any questions you had about seafood, food safety, or how much weight to gain. I especially hope it helped you manage your pregnancy with a smile on your face. And when your best friend calls to say she has "news," you can tell her you have just the thing to give her.

Notes

Introduction

1. *Pediatrics* Vol. 120 No. 6. December 2007, pp. 1247–1254 (doi:10.1542/peds.2007-0858).
2. Chatzi L, Torrent M, Romieu I, Garcia-Esteban R, Ferrer C, Vioque J, Kogevinas M, and Sunyer J. "Mediterranean Diet in pregnancy protective for wheeze and atopy in childhood." *Thorax*. Published online first: January 15, 2008. doi:10.1136/thx.2007.081745.

Trying for a Bump

1. American Society for Reproductive Medicine (ASRM). *Age and Fertility: A Guide for Patients*. ASRM, Birmingham, AL, 2003.
2. Chavarro JE et al. "Use of multivitamins, intake of B vitamins, and risk of ovulatory infertility." *Fertility and Sterility* 2007 Jul 9; 17624345.
3. "Huge Drop in Preterm Birth-Risk Among Women Taking Folic Acid One Year Before Conception," *March of Dimes News Desk* Jan 31, 2008. www.marchofdimes.com/aboutus/22684_28610.asp.
4. Chavaroo, JE, et al. "Iron intake and risk of ovulatory infertility." *Obstetrics & Gynecology* 108 (5): 1145–1152, November 2006.
5. *Journal of Agricultural and Food Chemistry*. 56 (4), 2008. 10.1021/jf073035s.
6. Chavarro JE et al. "A prospective study of dairy foods intake and anovulatory infertility." *Human Reproduction* pp. 1–8, 2007; doi:10.1093/humrep/dem019
7. "You are what your mother eats: Evidence for maternal preconception diet influencing foetal sex in humans." *Proceedings of the Royal Society* Vol. 275, Number 1643 / July 22, 2008, p. 1661–1668; doi: 10.1098/rspb.2008.0105
8. Chavarro et al. "Dietary fatty acid intakes and the risk of ovulatory infertility." *American Journal of Clinical Nutrition* Vol. 85, No. 1, 231–237, January 2007.

9. National Institute on Alcohol Abuse and Alcoholism of the National Institutes of Health. *National Institute on Alcohol Abuse and Alcoholism* No. 26 PH 352 October 1994. http://pubs.niaaa.nih.gov/publications/aa26.htm.

10. Bates GW. "American Society of Reproductive Medicine's Paper on Body Weight and Infertility." www.protectyourfertility.org/femalerisks.html#weight.

11. American Society for Reproductive Medicine Patient Fact Sheet on Stress and Infertility.

12. Society for Endocrinology Media Release. "Stress in pregnancy may affect the unborn child." May 31, 2007 (regarding research by Vivette Glover and Pampa Sarkar published in May 07 *Clinical Endocrinology* 66 (5), 636–640)

13. American Thoracic Society 2008 International Conference: Abstract A231. Presented May 18, 2008. *American Journal of Respiratory and Critical Care Medicine.* 2008; 177(suppl):A231.

14. ASRM Patient Fact Sheet On Diagnostic Testing For Male Factor Infertility, updated May 2008.

15. Sheynkin Y, et al. "Increase in scrotal temperature in laptop computer users." *Human Reproduction* 2005 20(2):452–455; doi:10.1093/humrep/deh616.

16. Agarwal A, et al. "Effect of cell phone usage on semen analysis in men attending infertility clinic: an observational study." *Fertility and Sterility* 2008 Jan; 89(1):124–8. Epub 2007 May 4.

17. Chavarro, et al. "Soy food and isoflavone intake in relation to semen quality parameters among men from an infertility clinic." *Human Reproduction* doi:10.1093/humrep/den243.

18. Soy serving size information from the Soy Foods Council.

19. Greco E, et al. "ICSI in case of sperm DNA damage: Beneficial effect of oral antioxidant treatment." *Human Reproduction* 2005 20(9): 2590–2594; doi:10.1093/humrep/dei091.

20. "Folate intake linked to genetic abnormalities in sperm." *UC Newsroom* www.universityofcalifornia.edu/news/article/17516.

21. Turk G, et al. "Effects of pomegranate juice consumption on sperm quality, spermatogenic cell density, antioxidant activity and testosterone level in male rats." *Clinical Nutrition* 2008 Apr; 27(2): 289–96. Epub 2008 Jan 28.

22. "Pomegranate juice may be good for the prostate and heart, reports the Harvard Men's Health Watch." *Medical News Today,* April 1, 2007.

23. E-mail interview with Dr. Maggie Somerall.

24. Curtis GB and Schuler J. *Your Pregnancy Week by Week, A Guide to Your Oral Health.* From Oral B.

Baby Bonuses and Momma Must-Haves

1. International Food Information Council and March of Dimes: Healthy Eating During Pregnancy, updated in 2005.

2. www.nal.usda.gov.

3. Coppen A, Bolander-Gouaille C. "Treatment of depression: Time to consider folic acid and vitamin B$_{12}$." *Journal of Psychopharmacology* 2005 Jan;19(1):59–65.

4. American Heart Association Fact Sheet on Homocysteine, Folic Acid, and Cardiovascular Disease.

5. *National Heart Lung and Blood Institute Diseases and Conditions Index,* Anemia.

6. March of Dimes Routine Prenatal Tests. www.marchofdimes.com/pnhec/159_519.asp.

7. Williams RD and Stehlin I. "Breast milk or formula: Making the right choice for your baby." U.S. Food and Drug Administration, *FDA Consumer Magazine*, updated June 1996. www.fda.gov/fdac/reprints/breastfed.html.

8. www.nal.usda.gov.

9. www.nal.usda.gov.

10. Hallberg L. "Does calcium interfere with iron absorption?" *American Journal of Clinical Nutrition* 1998 68: 3–4.

11. www.nal.usda.gov and National Turkey Federation.

12. *Pregnancy Food Guide* PDF from March of Dimes and Journal of the American College of Nutrition, Vol. 19, No. 90005, 528S–531S (2000).

13. Institute of Medicine, National Academy of Sciences. *Choline.* Dietary reference intakes for thiamin, riboflavin, niacin, vitamin B$_6$, folate, vitamin B$_{12}$, pantothenic acid, biotin, and choline. 1998.

14. USDA Database for the Choline Content of Common Foods, release two.

15. Xu et al. "Choline metabolism and risk of breast cancer in a population-based study." *Federation of American Societies for Experimental Biology Journal* 2008; 22: 2045–2052. www.pubmedcentral.nih.gov/articlerender.fcgi?tool=pubmed&pubmedid=18230680.

16. *Healthy Eating During Pregnancy*, Jan 2003. International Food Information Council Foundation and March of Dimes. www.ific.org/publications/brochures/pregnancybroch.cfm.

17. www.nal.usda.gov.

18. American Lung Association. State of the Air, 2008.

19. Bennett B. "The low-down on osteoporosis." *The NIH Word on Health*. December 2003.

20. www.nal.usda.gov.

21. www.nal.usda.gov.

22. NIH Office of Dietary Supplements, Fact Sheet on Vitamin B$_{12}$.

23. Casella EB. "Vitamin B$_{12}$ deficiency in infancy as a cause of developmental regression." *Brain and Development* Vol 27, Issue 8, December 2005, p. 592–594.

24. Institute of Medicine Table on Dietary Reference Intakes of Vitamins.

25. Institute of Medicine Table on Dietary Reference Intakes of Vitamins.

26. www.nal.usda.gov.

27. www.nal.usda.gov.

28. www.nal.usda.gov.

29. www.nal.usda.gov.
30. Northwestern University Feinberg School of Nutrition, Nutrition Fact Sheet on Iodine (online).
31. Public Health Nutrition. 2007 Dec; 10 (12A); 1532–9; discussion 1540–1.
32. Northwestern University Feinberg School of Nutrition, Nutrition Fact Sheet on Iodine (online).
33. Institute of Medicine Table on Dietary Reference Intakes of Vitamins.
34. www.nal.usda.gov.
35. Institute of Medicine Table on Dietary Reference Intakes of Vitamins.
36. www.nal.usda.gov.
37. National Institutes of Health Office of Dietary Supplements, Fact Sheet on Vitamin A and Carotenoids.
38. National Institutes of Health Office of Dietary Supplements, Fact Sheet on Vitamin A and Carotenoids.
39. Institute of Medicine Table on Dietary Reference Intakes of Vitamins www.iom.edu/Object.File/Master/7/294/0.pdf.
40. www.nal.usda.gov.
41. Institute of Medicine Table on Dietary Reference Intakes of Vitamins www.iom.edu/Object.File/Master/7/294/0.pdf.
42. www.nal.usda.gov.
43. Healthy Eating During Pregnancy, Jan 2003. International Food information Council Foundation and March of Dimes.

She's Gotta Have It

1. Pope JE, Skinner JD, Carruth BR. "Cravings and aversions of pregnant adolescents." *Journal of the American Dietetic Association* 1992; 92:1479–82.
2. Hook EB. "Dietary cravings and aversions during pregnancy." *American Journal of Clinical Nutrition* 1978; 31: 1355–62.
3. Tsegaye Demissie et al. "Food aversions and cravings during pregnancy: Prevalence and significance for maternal nutrition in Ethiopia." *United Nations University Press Food and Nutrition Bulletin,* Vol 19, Number 1.
4. Nordin S. "A longitudinal descriptive study of self-reported abnormal smell and taste perception in pregnant women." *Chemical Senses* Vol 29, 391–402, 2004.
5. American College of Obstetricians and Gynecologists Educational Pamphlet (online) AP001, Nutrition During Pregnancy. www.acog.org/publications/patient_education/bp001.cfm.

The Pregnancy Pantry

1. American Institute for Cancer Research. Finding nutrition fresh, frozen, and in cans, Enewsletter, November 2006. www.aicr.org/site/News2?abbr=pub_&page=NewsArticle&id=10727.

2. Willers S et al. "Maternal food consumption during pregnancy and the longitudinal development of childhood asthma." *American Journal of Respiratory and Critical Care Medicine* Vol 178. pp. 124–131 (2008).

What to Shelve for Nine Months

1. March of Dimes, Professionals & Researchers, Preconception Risk Reduction, Smoking During Pregnancy. http://search.marchofdimes.com/cgi-bin/MsmGo.exe?grab_id=6&page_id=13107200&query=smoking&hiword=smoking+.

2. American College of Obstetricians and Gynecologists, Pamphlet on Bleeding During Pregnancy.

3. March of Dimes, Professionals & Researchers, Preconception Risk Reduction, Smoking During Pregnancy. http://search.marchofdimes.com/cgi-bin/MsmGo.exe?grab_id=6&page_id=13107200&query=smoking&hiword=smoking+.

4. March of Dimes, Professionals & Researchers, Preconception Risk Reduction, Smoking During Pregnancy. http://search.marchofdimes.com/cgi-bin/MsmGo.exe?grab_id=6&page_id=13107200&query=smoking&hiword=smoking+.

5. www.smokefreeworld.com/usa.shtml.

6. March of Dimes, Professionals & Researchers, Preconception Risk Reduction, Drinking Alcohol During Pregnancy. http://search.marchofdimes.com/cgi-bin/MsmGo.exe?grab_id=6&page_id=11404800&query=alcohol&hiword=ALCOHOLIC+ALCOHOLISM+ALCOHOLS+alcohol+.

7. March of Dimes, Professionals & Researchers, Preconception Risk Reduction, Drinking Alcohol During Pregnancy. http://search.marchofdimes.com/cgi-bin/MsmGo.exe?grab_id=6&page_id=11404800&query=alcohol&hiword=ALCOHOLIC+ALCOHOLISM+ALCOHOLS+alcohol+.

8. Augustin J et al. "Alcohol retention in food preparation." *Journal of the American Dietetic Association* 92(4):486–488, 1992.

9. Kaiser Permanente Division of Research (2008, January 22). "Caffeine is linked to miscarriage risk, new study shows."

10. www.naturopathic-medicine.net/naturopathic/aromatherapy/aromatherapy-and-essential-oils.html.

11. *New Scientist* April 2004, based on study in *Early Human Development* Vol 76, p. 139.

12. Triche et al. "Chocolate consumption in pregnancy and reduced likelihood of preeclampsia." *Epidemiology.* 19(3):459–464, May 2008.

13. Letters to the Editor: "Effects of theobromine should be considered in future studies," *American Journal of Clinical Nutrition*, Vol. 82, No. 2, 486–487, August 2005.

14. www.nal.usda.gov, The Tea Council, www.wetplanet.com, and CSPI (Center for Science in the Public Interest).

15. FDA Issues Health Advisory about Certain Soft Cheese Made from Raw Milk, March 14, 2005. www.fda.gov/bbs/topics/news/2005/NEW01165.html.

16. Centers for Disease Control and Prevention, Preventing Health Risks. Association with Drinking Unpasteurized or Untreated Juice.

17. Kombucha mushroom tea cautions and concerns. Smart brewing tips by Ed Kasper Lac, acupuncturist, herbalist, and homeotoxicologist. Special concerns: Pregnant, children, and nursing.

18. U.S. Food and Drug Administration Center for Food Safety and Applied Nutrition. Food Safety for Moms-to-Be, August 24, 2005. www.cfsan.fda.gov/~pregnant/while.html.

19. U.S. Food and Drug Administration Center for Food Safety and Applied Nutrition. Food Safety for Moms-to-Be, August 24, 2005. www.cfsan.fda.gov/~pregnant/while.html.

20. U.S. Food and Drug Administration Center for Food Safety and Applied Nutrition. Food Safety for Moms-to-Be, August 24, 2005. www.cfsan.fda.gov/~pregnant/while.html.

21. "What you need to know about mercury in fish and shellfish. Advice for women who might become pregnant, women who are pregnant, nursing mothers, and young children." From the U.S. Food and Drug Administration and Environmental Protection Agency.

22. Burros M. "High mercury levels are found in tuna sushi." *New York Times*, January 23, 2008. www.nytimes.com/2008/01/23/dining/23sushi.html?_r=1&scp=1&sq=high%20levels%20of%20mercury%20in%20tuna&st=cse&oref=slogin.

23. "What you need to know about mercury in fish and shellfish. Advice for women who might become pregnant, women who are pregnant, nursing mothers, and young children." From the U.S. Food and Drug Administration and Environmental Protection Agency.

24. Fact sheet from Clemson University Home and Garden Information section and www.cfsan.fda.gov sheet on pathogens. http://hgic.clemson.edu/factsheets/HGIC3663.htm.

25. U.S. Department of Health and Human Services, "Sugar Substitutes: Americans opt for sweetness and lite." Updated February 2006. www.cfsan.fda.gov/~dms/fdsugar.html.

26. www.cfsan.fda.gov/~rbd/opa-g253.html.

27. "FDA issues midnight go-ahead for potentially harmful Stevia sweetener." *Center for Science in the Public Interest*, Dec 18, 2008

28. DerMarderosian A, Beutler J, eds. *Review of Natural Products*. St. Louis: Wolters Kluwer Health, 2004

29. Strandberg et al. "Preterm birth and licorice consumption during pregnancy." *American Journal of Epidemiology* 2002; 156:803–805.

30. From the Hershey's website: Licorice and glycyrrhizic acid.

31. Herb and drug safety chart, reprinted on Baby Centre, from *Herbs for a Healthy Pregnancy: From Conception to Childbirth* by Penelope Ody.

32. Conversation with Dawn Bierschwal, owner of Becoming Mom Spa in Mason, OH (513-770-6730).

33. Conversation with Dawn Bierschwal, owner of Becoming Mom Spa in Mason, OH (513-770-6730).

34. Conversation with Dawn Bierschwal, owner of Becoming Mom Spa in Mason, OH (513-770-6730).

35. "As retailers drop BPA, baby bottles get new scrutiny." *U.S. News & World Report*, April 22, 2008.

36. "Update: Toys "R" Us to phase out BPA baby bottles," *Washingtonpost.com*, April 21, 2008, and "Wal-Mart to pull bottles made with chemical BPA," *Washingtonpost.com*, April 18, 2008.

The Big O (Organic, That Is)

1. "Premature births may be linked to seasonal levels of pesticides and nitrates in surface water." Indiana University School of Medicine, May 2007.

2. "Organic milk is cream of the crop." Newcastle University Press Office, May 2008.

3. "Organic milk is cream of the crop." Newcastle University Press Office, May 2008.

4. USDA National Agricultural Library, Alternative Farming Systems Information Center, Organic Production/Organic Food: Information Access Tools, compiled by Mary V. Gold. Relevant text:

   What is organic food? Organic food is produced by farmers who emphasize the use of renewable resources and the conservation of soil and water to enhance environmental quality for future generations. Organic meat, poultry, eggs, and dairy products come from animals that are given no antibiotics or growth hormones. Organic food is produced without using most conventional pesticides; fertilizers made with synthetic ingredients or sewage sludge; bioengineering; or ionizing radiation. Before a product can be labeled "organic," a government-approved certifier inspects the farm where the food is grown to make sure the farmer is following all the rules necessary to meet USDA organic standards. Companies that handle or process organic food before it gets to your local supermarket or restaurant must be certified, too.

   Consumer Brochure, USDA National Organic Program, www.ams.usda.gov/nop/Consumers/brochure.html.

5. Environmental Working Group Shopper's Guide to Pesticides in Produce, www.foodnews.org.

Go Fish

1. "What you need to know about mercury in fish and shellfish. 2004 EPA and FDA advice for: Women who might become pregnant, women who are pregnant, nursing mothers, young children." www.cfsan.fda.gov/~dms/admehg3.html.

2. Interview with Steve Otwell, professor at the School of Food Science and Nutrition at the University of Florida in Gainesville.

3. "Mothers again urged to eat fish: Advisory at odds with FDA stance," October 4, 2007. www.washingtonpost.com/wp-dyn/content/article/2007/10/03/AR2007 100301278.html.

4. Hibbeln JR. "Maternal seafood consumption in pregnancy and neurodevelopmental outcomes in childhood (ALSPAC study): and observational cohort study." *The Lancet* 2007; 369: 578–85.

5. Mean and Percentiles for Usual Daily Intake of n-3 Docosahexaenoic Acid (22:6) (g), United States, CSFII (1994–1996, 1998).

6. International Food Information Council, "Fish and Your Health educational booklet"; www.nal.usda.gov.

7. Freeman M et al. "Omega-3 fatty acids: Evidence basis for treatment and future research in psychiatry." *The Journal of Clinical Psychiatry* 2006; 67: 1954–1967.

8. Hibbeln J. "Seafood consumption, the DHA content of mothers' milk and prevalence rates of postpartum depression: A cross-national, ecological analysis." *Journal of Affective Disorders* Vol. 69, 2002, pp. 15–29.

9. Freeman M et al. "Randomized dose-ranging pilot trial of omega-3 fatty acids for postpartum depression." *Acta Psychiatrica Scandinavica*, 2005: 1–5.

10. American Heart Association. "Fish and omega-3 fatty acids, AHA recommendation." www.americanheart.org/presenter.jhtml?identifier=4632.

11. Romieu I et al. "Maternal fish intake during pregnancy and atopy and asthma in infancy." *Clinical and Experimental Allergy* 2007; 37:518–525.

12. Oken E et al. "Maternal fish intake during pregnancy, blood mercury levels, and child cognition at age 3 years in a U.S. cohort." *American Journal of Epidemiology* 2008 167(10): 1171–1181; doi:10.1093/aje/kwn034.

13. U.S. Department of Health and Human Services and U.S. Environmental Protection Agency, "Mercury Levels in Commercial Fish and Shellfish," updated February 2006.

14. Monterey Bay Aquarium Seafood Watch. www.mbayaq.org/cr/cr_seafoodwatch/download.asp.

How to Deal When You're Meat-Free, Dairy-Free, or Wheat-Free

1. Vegetarian Times poll. www.prnewwire.com/cgi-bin/stories.pl?ACCT=104&STORY=/www/story/04-15-2008/0004792955&EDATE=.

2. www.nal.usda.gov.

3. www.nal.usda.gov.

4. www.nal.usda.gov, www.HorizonOrganic.com, and www.OikosOrganic.com.

5. National Digestive Diseases Information Clearinghouse (NDDIC) Fact Sheet on Celiac Disease. http://digestive.niddk.nih.gov/ddiseases/pubs/celiac.

6. "Celiac disease affects twice as many women." *Society for Women's Health Research* May 22, 2008. www.newswise.com/articles/view/541081.

7. Greer et al. "Effects of early nutritional interventions on the development of atopic disease in infants and children: The role of maternal dietary restriction, breast-feeding, timing of introduction of complementary foods, and hydrolyzed formulas." *Pediatrics* Vol. 121 No. 1 January 2008, pp. 183–191, doi:10.1542/peds.2007-3022. http://aap-policy.aappublications.org/cgi/content/abstract/pediatrics;121/1/183.

Belly Blues—Morning Sickness Survival Guide

1. Amelianova et al. "Prevalence and severity of nausea and vomiting of pregnancy and effect of vitamin supplementation." *Clinical and Investigative Medicine* 1999: 22(3): 106–10. www.nvp-volumes.org/p2_3.htm.
2. American College of Obstetricians and Gynecologists Pamphlet on Morning Sickness www.acog.org/publications/patient_education/bp126.cfm.
3. What to Expect website. www.whattoexpect.com/pregnancy/symptoms-and-solutions/metallic-taste.aspx.
4. Czeizel et al. "The effect of preconceptional multivitamin supplementation on the menstrual cycle." *Archives of Gynecology and Obstetrics* Vol 251, Number 4/July, 1992.
5. Amelianova et al. "Prevalence and severity of nausea and vomiting of pregnancy and effect of vitamin supplementation." *Clinical and Investigative Medicine* 1999: 22 (3): 106–10. www.nvp-volumes.org/p2_3.htm.
6. *American Journal of Obstetrics and Gynecology*, Vol 91, Issue 1, Jan 1998, pp. 78–81.
7. Grundy D. "Nausea and vomiting—an interdisciplinary approach." *Autonomic Neuroscience.* 2006 Oct 30; 129(1–2): 107–17. Epub 2006 Sep 1.
8. Baker L. "Morning sickness is linked to lower risk of breast cancer." *University of Buffalo Reporter.* July 12, 2007. www.buffalo.edu/reporter/vol38/vol38n43/articles/JaworowiczMorningSickness.html.
9. "Researchers discover how embryo attaches to the uterus." January 16, 2003 www.nichd.nih.gov/news/releases/embryo.cfm.
10. E-mail interview with Miriam Erick, MS, RD, CDE.
11. American Pregnancy Association Fact Sheet on Hyperemesis Gravidarum www.americanpregnancy.org/pregnancycomplications/hyperemesisgravidarum.html.

Burps, Farts, Heartburn, Bloating, and Other Good Times

1. Interview with Dr. Maggie Somerall.
2. American Pregnancy Association Fact Sheet on Heartburn. www.americanpregnancy.org/pregnancyhealth/heartburn.html.
3. Interview with Dr. Maggie Somerall.
4. Beano FAQs. www.beanogas.com/BeanoFAQs.aspx.
5. *Merck Manual of Women's and Men's Health*, p. 278.
6. National Digestive Diseases Information Clearinghouse Fact Sheet on Hemorrhoids. http://digestive.niddk.nih.gov/ddiseases/pubs/hemorrhoids/Hemorrhoids.pdf.

7. www.nal.usda.gov and www.allbran.com.
8. American College of Obstetricians and Gynecologists Patient Pamphlet on High Blood Pressure During Pregnancy. www.acog.org/publications/patient_education/bp034.cfm.
9. World's Healthiest Foods website. www.whfoods.com.
10. World's Healthiest Foods website. www.whfoods.com.
11. American Pregnancy Association Fact Sheet on Yeast Infections During Pregnancy. www.americanpregnancy.org/pregnancycomplications/yeastinfectionpreg.html.
12. American Pregnancy Association Fact Sheet on Urinary Tract Infections. www.americanpregnancy.org/pregnancycomplications/utiduringpreg.html.
13. American Pregnancy Association Fact Sheet on Urinary Tract Infections. www.americanpregnancy.org/pregnancycomplications/utiduringpreg.html.

"Does My Butt Look Fat?" and Other Weighty Questions

1. USDA information sheet on weight gain during pregnancy. www.nal.usda.gov/wic-works/Sharing_Center/MO/Weight_Gain.pdf.
2. "Weight gain in pregnancy linked to overweight in kids." Harvard Medical School Office of Public Affairs news release on Oken study.
3. Telephone interview with Dr. Emily Oken.
4. Reexamination of IOM Pregnancy Weight Guidelines. www.iom.edu/CMS/3788/48191.aspx.
5. Statistics Related to Overweight and Obesity, Weight-Control Information Network.
6. Kiel et al. "Gestational weight gain and pregnancy outcomes in obese women." *Obstetrics & Gynecology*; October 2007; 110(4): 759.
7. Chu SY et al. "Association between obesity during pregnancy and increased use of health care." *New England Journal of Medicine* Vol. 358: 1444–1453.
8. Interview with Dr. Maggie Somerall.
9. Artal R et al. "A lifestyle intervention of weight-gain restriction: diet and exercise in obese women with gestational diabetes mellitus." *Applied Physiology, Nutrition and Metabolism* 2007-06-01, Vol 32, pp. 596–601. ACOG Press Release on Guidance to Ob-gyns on Impact of Obesity During Pregnancy, 8/31/05.
10. *Planning Your Pregnancy and Birth, Third Edition.* American College of Obstetricians and Gynecologists.

Sweating for Two

1. Dunn A et al. "Exercise treatment for depression: Efficacy and dose response." *American Journal of Preventive Medicine*, Vol 28, Issue 1, Jan 2005, pp. 140–141.
2. Clapp JF 3d. "The course of labor after endurance exercise during pregnancy." *American Journal of Obstetrics & Gynecology* 1990; 163: 1799–805.

3. "Pregnancy link to active children." *BBC News* November 23, 2007. http://news.bbc.co.uk/1/hi/health/7107782.stm.

4. Ybarra O et al. "Mental exercising through simple socializing: social interaction promotes general cognitive functioning." *Personality and Social Psychology Bulletin* Vol. 34, No. 2, 248–259 (2008) DOI: 10.1177/0146167207310454.

5. American Pregnancy Association Fact Sheet on Premature Labor. www.american-pregnancy.org/labornbirth/prematurelabor.html.

6. ACOG Pamphlet on Exercise During Pregnancy. www.acog.org/publications/patient_education/bp119.cfm.

7. www.bikramyoga.com.

8. Interview with Dr. Marlene Reid, spokesperson for the American Podiatric Medical Association.

9. E-mail correspondence with Dr. Sarah Boyce Sawyer. www.healthyskinalabama.com/content.asp?id=127851.

10. ACOG Pamphlet on Exercise During Pregnancy. www.acog.org/publications/patient_education/bp119.cfm.

11. ACOG Pamphlet on Exercise During Pregnancy. www.acog.org/publications/patient_education/bp119.cfm.

12. ACOG Pamphlet on Exercise During Pregnancy. www.acog.org/publications/patient_education/bp119.cfm.

13. ACOG Pamphlet on Exercise During Pregnancy. www.acog.org/publications/patient_education/bp119.cfm.

14. Clapp JF 3d and Little KD. "Effect of recreational exercise on pregnancy weight gain and subcutaneous fat deposition." *Medicine and Science in Sports and Exercise* 1995; 27:170–7.

15. Pennick VE and Young G. "Interventions for preventing and treating pelvic and back pain in pregnancy." *Cochrane Database of Systematic Reviews* 1998, Issue 3. Art. No.: CD001139. DOI: 10.1002/14651858.CD001139.pub2.

16. www.saraivanhoe.com/flash/sara_i_yoga.html.

17. Mørkved S et al. "Pelvic floor muscle training during pregnancy to prevent urinary incontinence: A single-blind randomized controlled trial." *Obstetrics and Gynecology* 2003:101(2): 313–319.

18. ACOG Pamphlet on Exercise During Pregnancy. www.acog.org/publications/patient_education/bp119.cfm.

19. ACOG Pamphlet on Exercise During Pregnancy. www.acog.org/publications/patient_education/bp119.cfm.

When Things Get a Little Complicated

1. Retnakaran et al. "Ethnicity Modifies the Effect of Obesity on Insulin Resistance in Pregnancy: A Comparison of Asian, South Asian, and Caucasian Women," *The Journal of Clinical Endocrinology and Metabolism* Vol. 91, No. 1 93–97.

2. Lawrence J et al. "Trends in the prevalence of pre-existing diabetes and gestational diabetes mellitus among a racially/ethnically diverse population of pregnant women," 1999-2005. Kaiser Permanente study. *Diabetes Care* 31:899–904, 2008 DOI: 10.2337/dc07-2345.

3. ACOG Pamphlet on Gestational Diabetes. www.acog.org/publications/patient_education/bp051.cfm.

4. ACOG Pamphlet on Gestational Diabetes. www.acog.org/publications/patient_education/bp051.cfm.

5. National Library of Medicine Medline Plus Gestational Diabetes Fact Sheet. www.nlm.nih.gov/medlineplus/ency/article/000896.htm.

6. Bodnar et al. "Maternal vitamin D deficiency increases the risk of preeclampsia." *The Journal of Clinical Endocrinology & Metabolism* 2007; 92 (9): 3517–22.

7. Sharma JB, et al. "Effect of lycopene on pre-eclampsia and intra-uterine growth retardation in primigravidas." *The International Journal of Gynecology & Obstetrics* 2003; 81: 257–262.

8. "ACOG and high blood pressure during pregnancy." www.acog.org/publications/patient_education/bp034.cfm.

9. "Marcia Cross: Her happy new life." http://living.health.com/2008/04/21/marcia-cross-her-happy-new-life/.

10. "ACOG and high blood pressure during pregnancy." www.acog.org/publications/patient_education/bp034.cfm.

11. Smulian J et al. "Twin deliveries in the United States over three decades: An age-period-cohort analysis." *Obstetrics & Gynecology* 2004;104:278–285.

12. Martin J et al. "Births: Final data for 2003." *National Vital Statistics Report* Vol. 54, number 2, September 8, 2005.

13. Homburg et al. "The paradox of declining fertility but increasing twinning rates with advancing maternal age." *Human Reproduction* Advance Access published February 23, 2006.

14. Phenylketonuria. www.health.com/health/library/topic/0,,hw44745_hw44747,00.html.

Germ Patrol

1. U.S. Food and Drug Administration Center for Food Safety and Applied Nutrition, CFSAN/Office of Food Safety, Defense, and Outreach, August 24, 2005. Food Safety for Moms-to-Be, Information for Medical Professionals, Top 14 Foodborne Pathogens.

2. U.S. Food and Drug Administration Center for Food Safety and Applied Nutrition, CFSAN/Office of Food Safety, Defense, and Outreach, August 24, 2005. Food Safety for Moms-to-Be, Information for Medical Professionals, Top 14 Foodborne Pathogens.

3. U.S. Food and Drug Administration Center for Food Safety and Applied Nutrition, CFSAN/Office of Food Safety, Defense, and Outreach, August 24, 2005. Food Safety for Moms-to-Be, Information for Medical Professionals, Top 14 Foodborne Pathogens.

4. U.S. Food and Drug Administration Center for Food Safety and Applied Nutrition, CFSAN/Office of Food Safety, Defense, and Outreach, August 24, 2005. Food Safety for Moms-to-Be, Information for Medical Professionals, Top 14 Foodborne Pathogens.

5. U.S. Food and Drug Administration Center for Food Safety and Applied Nutrition, CFSAN/Office of Food Safety, Defense, and Outreach, August 24, 2005. Food Safety for Moms-to-Be, Information for Medical Professionals, Top 14 Foodborne Pathogens.

6. University of California, Division of Agriculture and Natural Resources research update, expanded research to target *E. coli* outbreaks. Issue Jan–Mar, 2007.

7. U.S. Food and Drug Administration Center for Food Safety and Applied Nutrition, CFSAN/Office of Food Safety, Defense, and Outreach, August 24, 2005. Food Safety for Moms-to-Be, Information for Medical Professionals, Top 14 Foodborne Pathogens.

8. Jordan Lin CT, Morales RA, and Ralston K. "Raw and undercooked eggs: A danger of salmonellosis." *Journal of Food Safety*, Jan–April 1997.

9. U.S. Food and Drug Administration Center for Food Safety and Applied Nutrition, CFSAN/Office of Food Safety, Defense, and Outreach, August 24, 2005. Food Safety for Moms-to-Be, Information for Medical Professionals, Top 14 Foodborne Pathogens.

10. Alabama Cooperative Extension System, Newsline. "Listeria: Craftier than first believed." February 10, 2004; U.S. Food and Drug Administration, FDA Statement, FDA issues health advisory about certain soft cheese made from raw milk. March 14, 2005.

11. National Center for Infectious Diseases, Respiratory and Enteric Viruses Branch, Norovirus: Food Handlers. What are noroviruses?

12. Centers for Disease Control and Prevention, Natural Disasters and Special Populations, Effect on Pregnant Women, Norovirus.

13. U.S. Food and Drug Administration Center for Food Safety and Applied Nutrition, CFSAN/Office of Food Safety, Defense, and Outreach, August 24, 2005. Food Safety for Moms-to-Be, Information for Medical Professionals, Top 14 Foodborne Pathogens.

14. Correspondence with Shelly Feist, executive director at the Partnership for Food Safety Education; www.fightbac.org.

15. U.S. Food and Drug Administration Center for Food Safety and Applied Nutrition, National Science Teachers Association, The A to Z. www.cfsan.fda.gov/~dms/a2z-b.html.

16. www.fightbac.org.

17. www.fightbac.org.

18. www.fightbac.org.

19. Kravetz JD and Federman DG. Toxoplasmosis in pregnancy. *American Journal of Medicine*, 2005 Mar; 118 (3): 212–6.

20. National Restaurant Association report on meal consumption behavior, 2000.

21. Research Report: Cubicle Culture Survey, September 8, 2005.

22. "First in-office study dishes the dirt on desks, researchers find average desk harbors 400 times more bacteria than average toilet seat." 4, 15, 2002. www.disinfecttoprotect.com/downloads/Office-Study.pdf.

23. http://living.health.com/2008/03/12/the-germiest-places-in-america.
24. http://living.health.com/2008/03/12/the-germiest-places-in-america.

Belly in the Kitchen

1. Phone interview with Dr Marlene Reid.
2. Phone interview with Dr Marlene Reid.
3. Phone interview with Dr Marlene Reid.
4. Healthline. "Bodily changes during pregnancy, reviewed February 2006." www.healthline.com/yodocontent/pregnancy/bodily-changes-during.html.

Momma Munchies

1. Nutrition information: www.nal.usda.gov and Food Processor from ESHA Research.
2. Helmenstine, AM. "Does eating turkey make you sleepy? Tryptophan and carbohydrate chemistry." *About.com.* http://chemistry.about.com/od/holidaysseasons/a/tiredturkey.htm.

The Milk Factory and Beyond

1. ACOG Educational Bulletin Number 258, July 2000: *Breast-feeding: Maternal and Infant Aspects*
2. Wolk M. "Weight loss while breast-feeding." *Leaven* Vol. 33 No. 5, October-November 1997, p. 115.
3. Institute of Medicine, Dietary Reference Intakes for Vitamins; Institute of Medicine, Dietary Reference Intakes for Minerals.
4. Kimata H. "Laughter elevates the levels of breast milk melatonin." *Journal of Psychosomatic Research* Vol. 62, Issue 6, pp. 699–702.
5. ACOG Pamphlet on Breast-feeding Your Baby. www.acog.org/publications/patient_education/bp029.cfm.
6. Dewey K. and McCrory M. "Effects of dieting and physical activity on pregnancy and lactation." *American Journal of Clinical Nutrition* 1994; 59(Suppl.): 446S–59S.
7. Lovelady C et al. "Lactation performance of exercising women." *American Journal of Clinical Nutrition* 1990; 52: 103–1.
8. *Losing weight after pregnancy: Diet and exercise better than diet alone.* John Wiley & Sons, Inc. (2007, July 18).

Index

About the Author

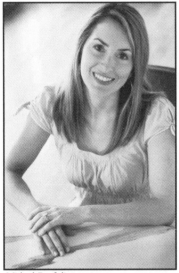

Michael Bonfigli

Frances Largeman-Roth, RD, is the senior food and nutrition editor at *Health* magazine. Frances earned her undergraduate degree from Cornell University and completed her dietetic internship at Columbia University in New York. She has had the opportunity to work with top chefs and food personalities, putting a healthier spin on recipes from Jamie Oliver, Mark Bittman, Emily Luchetti, Gale Gand, Rick Bayless, and Bobby Flay, among others. Frances is a member of the American Dietetic Association and the International Association of Culinary Professionals. Frances is a frequent guest on national TV, including appearances on the *Today Show, Good Morning America, The Early Show,* and *Fox & Friends.*

She lives in Brooklyn, New York, with her husband Jon, their daughter, and their flat-coated retriever Millie. Visit her at www.franceslargemanroth.com.

Feed the Belly
Seven-Day Eating Plan

So, the first trimester is over, and now you're into eating and growing mode.

Just like before you were with child, not every day of your pregnancy will be a perfect day, nutritionally or otherwise. There's the morning sickness to deal with, hectic schedules, and trips to the doctor, but on days that you can muster it, try to eat as this eating plan suggests as often as possible. This is the gold standard, kind of like exercising every day for at least forty-five minutes.

Don't think that you have to make each and every recipe in the plan. Just use them as a guide for what to choose and how much to eat overall. Also, don't feel constrained by the order in which I've listed the meals. You can have Monday's late-morning snack on Friday afternoon or eat breakfast for dinner, if that's your thing.

You'll see that I've included three snacks a day, plus a little something for when you get up (or when you're still in bed, trying to get your stomach under control). If you're not feeling up to it, it's fine to skip a snack. Just don't go longer than three to four hours without eating. And if you feel perfectly fine when you wake up, you won't need the stomach-settling nibble. If you end up eating dinner late—say, around 8 to 9 p.m.—you probably won't want to wait until later to have the evening snack, because it might give you heartburn. Just tack it onto dinner, or eat it when you come home from work.

I'm assuming that you were eating somewhere around 1,800 to 2,000 calories a day before you were pregnant. If you add 300 calories to that, you end up somewhere between 2,100 and 2,300, which is approximately what each day's menu includes.

This plan is perfect for your second and third trimester; if you'd like to follow it for your first trimester, just drop one or two of the snacks. When you're breast-feeding, you may need to add another 200-calorie snack. If you're a mom carrying multiples, you'll need to add more calories depending on your doctor's recommendation.

Each day on the plan is packed with baby-building protein (at least 92 g) and an average of 37 g fiber, 1,223 mg calcium, and 288 mcg folic acid (your prenatal multi will make up the rest). Grab your fork and dig in!

Monday

First thing in the morning, if you're nauseous:

3 whole-wheat crackers

Breakfast:

½ cup dry oatmeal (steel cut is ideal, but low-sugar instant is fine), prepared

½ cup organic blueberries, fresh or frozen

1 cup organic 1% or soy milk

1 ounce roasted almonds, unsalted

Late-morning snack:

1 medium orange

1 low-fat organic cheese stick

Lunch:

Mediterranean Barley Salad (page 213)

1 4-ounce grilled or roasted chicken breast

1 cup green grapes

Water

Mid-afternoon snack:

1 4-ounce serving all-natural chocolate pudding

1 organic apple

Dinner:

Ginger-Glazed Salmon (page 201)

1 cup brown rice

Spinach and Pear Salad with Pomegranate Dressing (page 211)

Water

Evening snack:

Better Than Elvis Milkshake (page 157)

Calories 2,272; Fat 75 g (Sat 14 g, Mono 24 g, Poly 17 g); Cholesterol 188 mg; Protein 120 g; Carbohydrate 299 g; Fiber 39 g; Iron 14 mg; Sodium 1,611 mg; Calcium 1,164 mg; Folic Acid 242 mcg; Vitamin C 154 mg

Tuesday

First thing in the morning, if you're nauseous:

¼ cup dry cereal, such as Barbara's Shredded Spoonfuls

Breakfast:

1 cup low-fat vanilla organic yogurt topped with ½ cup Hippie-Chick Granola (page 180) and 1 cup fresh raspberries

6 ounces grapefruit juice fortified with DHA

Late-morning snack:

1 organic pear

1 organic low-fat string cheese stick

1 4-inch whole-wheat pita

6 ounces orange juice with added calcium and vitamin D

Lunch:

Roasted Fall Vegetable Soup (page 219)

1 whole-wheat roll

1 1-ounce slice of Gruyère cheese

1 cup baby carrots

Water

Mid-afternoon snack:

4 graham crackers with 2 tablespoons natural peanut butter

8 ounces organic 1% milk

Dinner:

Alisa's Taco Salad with Yogurty Salsa (page 236)

1 1-ounce serving blue corn tortilla chips

Love That Bump Lemonade (page 252)

Evening snack:

Nana-Berry Smoothie (page 249)

Calories 2,302; Fat 69 g (Sat 20 g, Mono 17 g, Poly 5 g); Cholesterol 149 mg; Protein 105 g; Carbohydrate 339 g; Fiber 42 g; Iron 14 mg; Sodium 2,402 mg; Calcium 2,111 mg; Folic Acid 353 mcg; Vitamin C 325 mg

Wednesday

First thing in the morning, if you're nauseous:

3 stoned-wheat crackers

Breakfast:

Renée's Orange Creamsicle (page 250)

1 slice whole-wheat toast

1 tablespoon natural peanut butter

Late morning snack:

1 6-ounce serving organic low-fat vanilla yogurt

1 ounce walnut halves (about 14)

1 cup organic blueberries, fresh or frozen

Lunch:

Everything but the Kitchen Sink Frittata (page 204)

Green Salad

> 2 cups field greens, ½ cup cherry toma-
> toes, 2 tablespoons balsamic vinaigrette
> dressing fortified with omega-3, such
> as Spectrum

Gingery Watermelon Liquado (page
250)

Mid-afternoon snack:

2 tablespoons store-bought hummus

1 cup baby carrots

1 cup jicama or celery, sliced into sticks

Belly Tip
If you can't make
the frittata yourself or
find one at a restaurant,
go for an omelet packed
with veggies instead.

Belly Tip
You can order something similar at a Thai restaurant. Just
ask for the regular pad Thai
with less sauce (which
means less sodium)
and extra shrimp.

Dinner:

Pregnancy Pad Thai (page 241)

Sesame-Ginger Green Beans (page 247)

Water

1 large pear, quartered

Evening snack:

Sweet Baby Bread Pudding

8 ounces 1% milk

Calories 2,189; Fat 75 g (Sat 13 g, Mono 13 g, Poly 19 g); Cholesterol 350 mg; Protein 92 g; Carbohydrate 309 g; Fiber 43 g; Iron 15 mg; Sodium 2,484 mg; Calcium 1,288 mg; Folic Acid 292 mcg; Vitamin C 204 mg

Thursday

First thing in the morning, if you're nauseous:

3 whole-grain crackers, such as Kashi

Breakfast:

Mornin' Sunshine Parfait (page 170)

1 slice whole-wheat toast

1 tablespoon almond butter

1 teaspoon honey

6 ounces pomegranate juice (such as POM)

Late-morning snack:

Fresh Fruit with Creamy Yo-Co Dip (page 175)

Lunch:

Avocado and Swiss Veggie Delight

> Cook a veggie burger in a skillet on the stove or in the microwave. Melt a slice of Swiss cheese on top of the burger. Meanwhile, toast 2 slices of whole-wheat bread. Transfer the veggie burger to one slice of bread. Top with 1 cup of arugula leaves, ½ cup avocado slices, and ⅓ cup peeled cucumber slices. Top with the other slice of bread, cut in half, and serve.

Mango-Pineapple Crush (page 253)

Mid-afternoon snack:

2 Morning, Noon, and Night Nut Clusters (page 182)

1 Asian pear

Belly Tip

These clusters are amazing, but if you can't make them, try the ones from TrueNorth. www.truenorth snacks.com

8 ounces organic 1% milk

Dinner:

Pesto Pizza Pie (page 233)

1½ cups steamed broccoli rabe or broccoli

Water

Evening snack:

Papaya Blue Lagoon (page 254)

Calories 2,230; Fat 82 g (Sat 27 g, Mono 26 g, Poly 9 g); Cholesterol 80 mg; Protein 90 g; Carbohydrate 306 g; Fiber 35 g; Iron 11 mg; Sodium 2,089 mg; Calcium 1,598 mg; Folic Acid 322 mcg; Vitamin C 271 mg

Friday

First thing in the morning, if you're nauseous:

1 graham cracker

Breakfast:

6 ounces raspberry kefir, preferably organic

1 cup raspberries

¼ cup roasted unsalted almonds

Late-morning snack:

Baby on Board Banana Bread (page 179) or a snack bar formulated for pregnancy (see suggestions on page 142)

6 ounces ruby-red grapefruit juice

Lunch:

Farfalle with Edamame and Pecorino (page 224)

Arugula-Apple Salad

> Mix together 1 cup arugula, 1 cup sliced apples, and 1 tablespoon light Italian dressing.

Water

Mid-afternoon snack:

All-Purpose Veggie Dip (page 232)

½ cup halved radishes

½ cup sugar snap peas

½ cup celery sticks

Belly Tip

If you're in an urban area where there are lots of lunch places with a salad or pasta bar, you can make something similar to the farfalle using spiral or penne pasta, a little Parmesan cheese, and peas.

Dinner:

Momma's Meatloaf (page 194)

Brocco Mac and Cheese (page 222)

Water

Evening snack:

2 Pucker Up Mini Lemon Tartlets (page 163)

8 ounces organic 1% milk

Calories 2,231; Fat 77 g (Sat 27 g, Mono 20 g, Poly 7 g); Cholesterol 351 mg; Protein 102 g; Carbohydrate 297 g; Fiber 27 g; Iron 16 mg; Sodium 2,351 mg; Calcium 1,519 mg; Folic Acid 385 mcg; Vitamin C 145 mg

Saturday

First thing in the morning, if you're nauseous:

¼ cup dry corn flakes

Breakfast:

Huevos Rancheros Wrap (page 237)

6 ounces orange juice, fortified with calcium and vitamin D

Late-morning snack:

Fruity Booty Salad (page 176)

Lunch:

Warm Fig Salad with Pecans (page 215)

1 organic apple

Water

Mid-afternoon snack:

1 toasted whole-grain English muffin with 2 tablespoons natural peanut butter, topped with banana slices (about ½ banana)

Dinner:

Baked Mediterranean Tilapia (page 200)

1 cup brown rice

Roasted Spring Asparagus (page 225)

Water

Evening snack:

Oh! Susannah Chocolate Maltshake (page 162)

Calories 2,278; Fat 78 g (Sat 15, Mono 21 g, Poly 6); Cholesterol 409 mg; Protein 106 g; Carbohydrate 306 g; Fiber 42 g; Iron 13 mg; Sodium 2,193 mg; Calcium 881 mg; Folic Acid 215 mcg; Vitamin C 275 mg

Sunday

First thing in the morning, if you're nauseous:

Oh, Baby! Breakfast Cookie (page 183) or 18 pretzel snaps

Breakfast:

Oatmeal Brulée (page 169)

2 tablespoons chopped walnuts (sprinkle on top of oatmeal)

6 ounces pomegranate juice

Late-morning snack:

Chunky Monkey Muffin (page 158)

6 ounces organic chocolate soy milk

Lunch:

Tofu Wrap

> Slice 4 ounces extra firm tofu; set aside. Place a whole-wheat tortilla on a cutting board or large plate. Add the tofu to the center of the tortilla and sprinkle with 1 teaspoon paprika. Add ¼ cup sliced avocado and some chopped lettuce and tomato. Fold in the sides and top of wrap, and roll up toward you. Cut in half and serve.

Water

Mid-afternoon snack:

1 5.3-ounce container plain fat-free Greek yogurt (such as Fage or Oikos) mixed with ½ cup sliced organic strawberries and 1 tablespoon wheat germ

Dinner:

Lemony Chicken with Capers (page 190)

Confetti Rice Salad (page 208)

Mean Greens and Beans (page 228)

Water

Evening snack:

Peach and Blackberry Crumble (page 177)

6 ounces organic 1% milk

Calories 2,211; Fat 73 g (Sat 18 g, Mono 17 g, Poly 13 g); Cholesterol 140 mg; Protein 111 g; Carbohydrate 288 g; Fiber 33 g; Iron 16 mg; Sodium 1,790 mg; Calcium 1,414 mg; Folic Acid 210 mcg; Vitamin C 196 mg